Atrial Fibrillation Ablation, 2011 Update

T0176433

Atrial Fibrillation Ablation, 2011 Update

THE STATE OF THE ART BASED ON THE VENICECHART INTERNATIONAL CONSENSUS DOCUMENT

Edited by

Andrea Natale, MD, FACC, FESC, FHRS
Texas Cardiac Arrhythmia Institute
St. David's Medical Center, Austin, TX, USA

Antonio Raviele, MD, FESC, FHRS
Cardiovascular Department
Arrhythmia Center & Center for Atrial Fibrillation
Dell'Angelo Hospital, Venice-Mestre, Italy

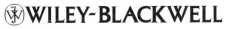
A John Wiley & Sons, Ltd., Publication

This edition first published 2011, © 2011 by John Wiley & Sons, Ltd.

Wiley-Blackwell is an imprint of John Wiley & Sons, formed by the merger of Wiley's global Scientific, Technical and Medical business with Blackwell Publishing.

Registered office: John Wiley & Sons, Ltd, The Atrium, Southern Gate, Chichester, West Sussex, PO19 8SQ, UK

Editorial offices: 9600 Garsington Road, Oxford, OX4 2DQ, UK
The Atrium, Southern Gate, Chichester, West Sussex, PO19 8SQ, UK
111 River Street, Hoboken, NJ 07030-5774, USA

For details of our global editorial offices, for customer services and for information about how to apply for permission to reuse the copyright material in this book please see our website at www.wiley.com/wiley-blackwell.

The right of the author to be identified as the author of this work has been asserted in accordance with the UK Copyright, Designs and Patents Act 1988.

All rights reserved. No part of this publication may be reproduced, stored in a retrieval system, or transmitted, in any form or by any means, electronic, mechanical, photocopying, recording or otherwise, except as permitted by the UK Copyright, Designs and Patents Act 1988, without the prior permission of the publisher.

Designations used by companies to distinguish their products are often claimed as trademarks. All brand names and product names used in this book are trade names, service marks, trademarks or registered trademarks of their respective owners. The publisher is not associated with any product or vendor mentioned in this book. This publication is designed to provide accurate and authoritative information in regard to the subject matter covered. It is sold on the understanding that the publisher is not engaged in rendering professional services. If professional advice or other expert assistance is required, the services of a competent professional should be sought.

The contents of this work are intended to further general scientific research, understanding, and discussion only and are not intended and should not be relied upon as recommending or promoting a specific method, diagnosis, or treatment by physicians for any particular patient. The publisher and the author make no representations or warranties with respect to the accuracy or completeness of the contents of this work and specifically disclaim all warranties, including without limitation any implied warranties of fitness for a particular purpose. In view of ongoing research, equipment modifications, changes in governmental regulations, and the constant flow of information relating to the use of medicines, equipment, and devices, the reader is urged to review and evaluate the information provided in the package insert or instructions for each medicine, equipment, or device for, among other things, any changes in the instructions or indication of usage and for added warnings and precautions. Readers should consult with a specialist where appropriate. The fact that an organization or Website is referred to in this work as a citation and/or a potential source of further information does not mean that the author or the publisher endorses the information the organization or Website may provide or recommendations it may make. Further, readers should be aware that Internet Websites listed in this work may have changed or disappeared between when this work was written and when it is read. No warranty may be created or extended by any promotional statements for this work. Neither the publisher nor the author shall be liable for any damages arising herefrom.

Library of Congress Cataloging-in-Publication Data is available for this title

A catalogue record for this book is available from the British Library.

This book is published in the following electronic formats: ePDF 9781119963837; Wiley Online Library 9781119963868; ePub 9781119963844; Mobi 9781119963851

Set in 9.5/12pt Palatino by Aptara® Inc., New Delhi, India

1   2011

Contents

This initiative has been made possible thanks to an unrestricted educational grant from

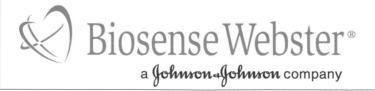

Preface

This book represents the extended version of the VeniceChart International Consensus Document on Atrial Fibrillation Ablation, 2011 Update, and includes the recent technological developments and progress on atrial fibrillation (AF) since our last edition. AF ablation has become a well-etablished, widespread treatment not only for patients with paroxysmal AF but also for patients with persistent and long-lasting persistent AF and is recognized by the most recent European and American guidelines on AF management.

As the list of contributors shows, many renowned experts have contributed to the preparation of the VeniceChart International Consensus Document and to the realization of this book. We are deeply indebted to all of them because without their enthusiasm and personal effort this volume would not have been possible. We also wish to acknowledge the unparalleled editorial work of Nick Godwin, Cathryn Gates, and Elisabeth Dodds of Wiley-Blackwell Publishers, as well as the invaluable dedication and assistance of Rita Reggiani, Raffaella Pieri, and Ludovica Fontana of Adria Congrex. Our heartfelt thanks go to our colleagues at the Texas Cardiac Arrhythmia Institute, in Austin, Texas, and at Ospedale Dell'Angelo, in Venice-Mestre, for the preparation and realization of both the VeniceChart International Consensus Document and the VeniceArrhythmias 2011 Workshop. In particular, we thank Drs Aldo Bonso, David J. Burkhardt, Andrea Corrado, Luigi Di Biase, Gianni Gasparini, Franco Giada, Michela Madalosso, Antonio Rossillo, Pasquale Santangeli, and Sakis Themistoclakis.

Last but not least, our gratitude goes to our families, without whose patience and continuous support we could not have accomplished this task. We are profoundly thankful to our wives, Carmen and Marina, our children, Francesca, Michele, Veronica, Eleonora, and grandchild Edoardo.

Andrea Natale
Antonio Raviele

List of contributors

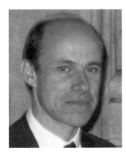

Pedro Adragao, MD
Cardiology Department
Hospital Santa Cruz
Carnaxide, Portugal

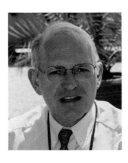

Etienne Aliot, MD
Cardio-vascular Diseases Department
CHU de Brabois,
Vandoeuvre-lès-Nancy, France

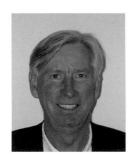

Maurits Allessie, MD
Cardiovascular Research Institute Maastricht
Maastricht, The Netherlands

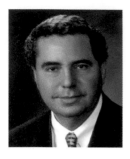

Charles Antzelevitch, MD
Masonic Medical Research Laboratory
Utica, NY, USA

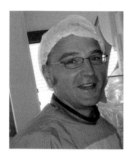

Thomas Arentz, MD
Rhythmology Department
Herz-Zentrum
Bad Krozingen, Germany

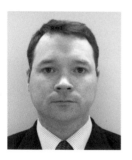

Conor Barrett, MD
Cardiac Arrhythmia Service
Massachusetts General Hospital
Boston, MA, USA

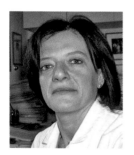

Cristina Basso, MD
Cardiovascular Pathology Department
University of Padua Medical School
Padua, Italy

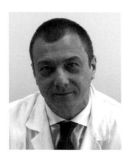

Stefano Benussi, MD
Cardiac Surgery Department
San Raffaele Hospital
Milan, Italy

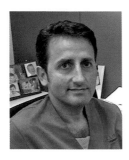

Antonio Berruezo, MD
Cardiology Department
Clinic Hospital
Barcelona, Spain

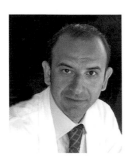

Emanuele Bertaglia, MD
Cardiology Department
ULSS 13 Mirano
Mirano, Italy

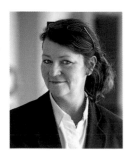

Carina Blomström-Lundqvist, MD
Cardiology Department
University Hospital in Uppsala
Uppsala, Sweden

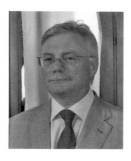

Aldo Bonso, MD
Cardiovascular Department
Dell'Angelo Hospital
Venice-Mestre, Italy

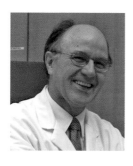

Johannes Brachmann, MD
Cardiology Department
II Med Klinik Klinikum Coburg
Coburg, Germany

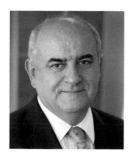

Josep Brugada, MD
Cardiology Department
Thorax Institute, Clinic of Barcelona
Barcelona, Spain

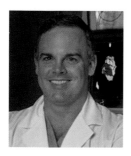

David J. Burkhardt, MD
Texas Cardiac Arrhythmia Institute
St. David's Medical Center
Austin, TX, USA

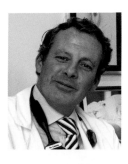

José A. Cabrera, MD
Arrhythmia Unit, Cardiology Department
Quirón Hospital, Universidad Europea de Madrid
Madrid, Spain

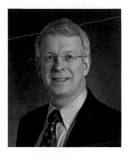

Hugh Calkins, MD
Cardiology and Electrophysiology Department
The Johns Hopkins Hospital
Baltimore, MD, USA

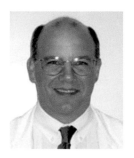

David Callans, MD
Cardiovascular Disease Department
Hospital of the University of Pennsylvania
Philadelphia, PA, USA

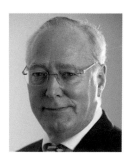

A. John Camm, MD
Cardiac and Vascular Sciences
St. George's Hospital Medical School
London, UK

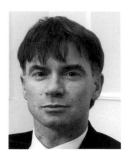

Riccardo Cappato, MD
Electrophysiology Department
Policlinico S. Donato
San Donato Milanese, Italy

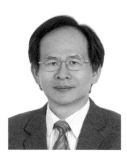

Shih-Ann Chen, MD
Cardiology Department
Veterans General Hospital
Taipei, Taiwan

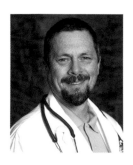

Stuart J. Connolly, MD
Cardiology Department
McMaster University
Hamilton, ON, Canada

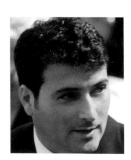

Andrea Corrado, MD
Cardiology Department
Dell'Angelo Hospital
Venice-Mestre, Italy

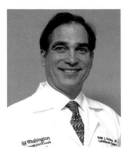

Ralph Damiano Jr., MD
Cardiothoracic Surgery Department
Washington University in St. Louis-School of Medicine
St. Louis, MO, USA

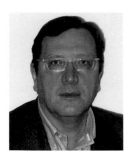

Roberto De Ponti, MD
Cardiology Department
Circolo Hospital and Macchi Foundation
Varese, Italy

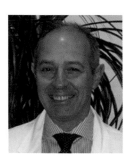

Paolo Della Bella, MD
Cardiology Department
San Raffaele Hospital
Milan, Italy

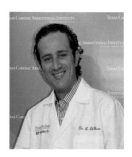

Luigi Di Biase, MD
Texas Cardiac Arrhythmia Institute
St. David's Medical Center
Austin, TX, USA

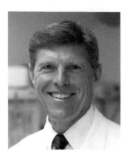

Paul Dorian, MD
Cardiology Department
St. Michael's Hospital
Toronto, ON, Canada

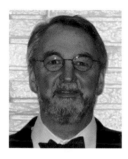

James R. Edgerton, MD
Cardiothoracic Surgery Department
The Heart Hospital
Dallas, TX, USA

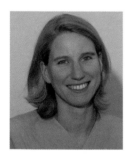

Sabine Ernst, MD
National Heart and Lung Institute
Royal Brompton and Harefield Hospital
Imperial College
London, UK

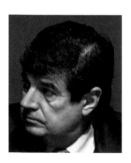

Jeronimo Farré, MD
Cardiology Department
Jiménez Díaz-Capio Foundation
Madrid, Spain

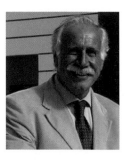

Fiorenzo Gaita, MD
Internal Medicine Department
University of Turin
Turin, Italy

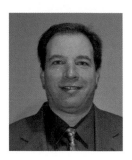

Edward B. Gerstenfeld, MD
Cardiac Electrophysiology Department
University of California
San Francisco, CA, USA

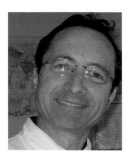

Michel Haïssaguerre, MD
Cardiology Department
Hôpital Haut-Lévêque, CHU de Bordeaux
Bordeaux, France

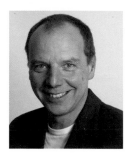

Gerhard Hindricks, MD
Herzzentrum
Leitender Arzt Universität Leipzig
Leipzig, Germany

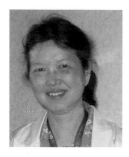

Siew Y. Ho, MD
Cardiac Morphology Department
Royal Brompton Hospital
Imperial College, London, UK

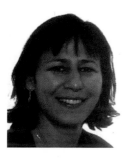

Mélèze Hocini, MD
Cardiology Department
Hôpital Haut-Lévêque, CHU de Bordeaux
Bordeaux, France

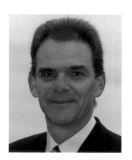

Stefan H. Hohnloser, MD
Electrophysiology Department
J.W. Goethe University
Frankfurt, Germany

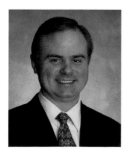

Rodney P. Horton, MD
Texas Cardiac Arrhythmia Institute
St. David's Medical Center
Austin, TX, USA

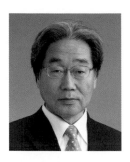

Yoshito Iesaka, MD
Tsuchiura Kyodo Hospital
Tsuchiura City, Japan

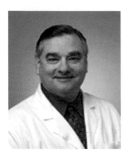

Warren M. Jackman, MD
Heart Rhythm Institute
Oklahoma City, OK, USA

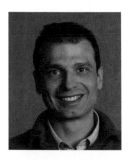

Pierre Jaïs, MD
Cardiology Department
Hôpital Haut-Lévêque, CHU de Bordeaux
Bordeaux, France

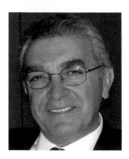

José Jalife, MD
University of Michigan
Ann Arbor, MI, USA

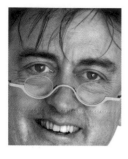

Luc J. Jordaens, MD
Thoraxcenter, Clinical Electrophysiology Department
Erasmus MC
Rotterdam, The Netherlands

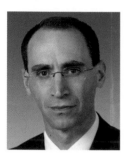

Jonathan M. Kalman, MD
Cardiology Department
Royal Melbourne and Western Hospitals
Melbourne, Australia

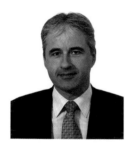

Josef Kautzner, MD
Cardiology Department
Institute for Clinical and Experimental Medicine
Prague, Czech Republic

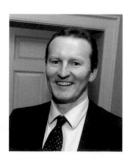

David Keane, MD
Cardiology Department
St. Vincent's University Hospital
Dublin, Ireland

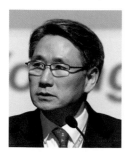

Young-Hoon Kim, MD
Cardiology and Electrophysiology Department
Korea University Medical Center
Seoul, South Korea

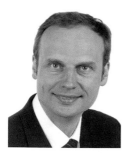

Paulus Kirchhof, MD
School of Clinical & Experimental Medicine
University of Birmingham
Birmingham, UK

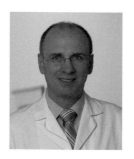

Hans Kottkamp, MD
Herz-Zentrum
Hirslanden Clinic
Zürich, Switzerland

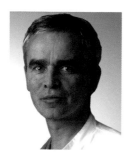

Karl H. Kuck, MD
Cardiology Department
Asklepios Klinik St. Georg
Hamburg, Germany

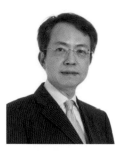

Chu-Pak Lau, MD
Cardiology Department
University of Hong Kong-Queen Mary Hospital
Hong Kong

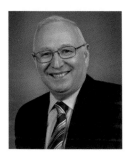

Samuel Lévy, MD
Cardiology Department
CHU Hôpital Nord
Marseille, France

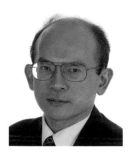

Gregory Y.H. Lip, MD
University Department of Medicine
City Hospital
Birmingham, UK

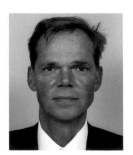

Jos G. Maessen, MD
Cardiothoracic Surgery Department
University of Maastricht
Maastricht, The Netherlands

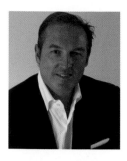

Helmut Mair, MD
Cardiac Surgery Department
University of Munich
Munich, Germany

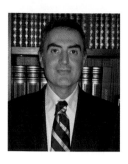

Domenico Mangino, MD
Cardiovascular Department
Dell'Angelo Hospital
Venice-Mestre, Italy

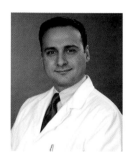

Moussa Mansour, MD
Cardiac Arrhythmia Department
Massachusetts General Hospital
Boston, MA, USA

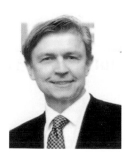

Francis E. Marchlinski, MD
Cardiovascular Division
Hospital of the University of Pennsylvania
Philadelphia, PA, USA

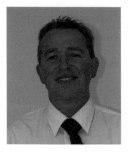

José L. Merino, MD
Cardiology Department
La Paz University Hospital
Madrid, Spain

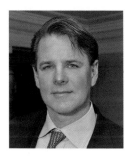

Gregory F. Michaud, MD
Center for Advanced Management of Atrial Fibrillation
Brigham and Women's Hospital
Boston, MA, USA

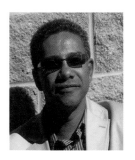

Carlos A. Morillo, MD
Arrhythmia & Pacing Department
Hamilton General Hospital
Hamilton, ON, Canada

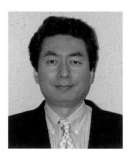

Hiroshi Nakagawa, MD
Heart Rhythm Institute
University of Oklahoma Health Sciences Center
Oklahoma City, OK, USA

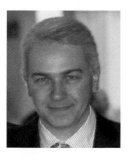

Andrea Natale, MD
Texas Cardiac Arrhythmia Institute
St. David's Medical Center
Austin, TX, USA

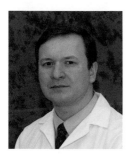

Hakan Oral, MD
Cardiovascular Medicine Department
University of Michigan
Ann Arbor, MI, USA

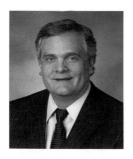

Douglas L. Packer, MD
Heart Rhythm Services
Mayo Clinic Health Systems/St. Mary's Hospital
Rochester, NY, USA

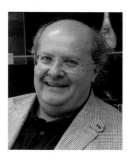

Carlo Pappone, MD
Arrhythmology Department
Villa Maria Cecilia Hospital
Cotignola, Italy

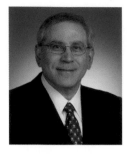

Eric N. Prystowsky, MD
Clinical Electrophysiology Laboratory
St. Vincent Indianapolis Hospital
Indianapolis, IN, USA

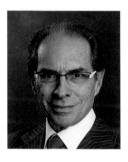

Antonio Raviele, MD
Cardiovascular Department
Arrhythmia Center & Center for Atrial Fibrillation
Dell'Angelo Hospital
Venice-Mestre, Italy

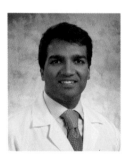

Vivek Y. Reddy, MD
Cardiac Arrhythmia Department
The Zena and Michael A. Wiener Cardiovascular Institute
New York, NY, USA

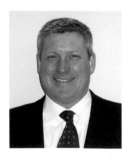

Matthew Reynolds, MD
Beth Israel Deaconess Medical Center
Harvard Clinical Research Institute
Boston, MA, USA

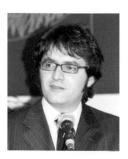

Antonio Rossillo, MD
Cardiovascular Department
Dell'Angelo Hospital
Venice-Mestre, Italy

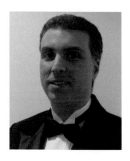

Eduardo Saad, MD
Center for Atrial Fibrillation
Pro-Cardiaco Hospital
Rio de Janeiro, Brazil

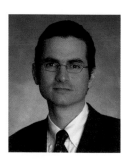

Javier E. Sanchez, MD
Texas Cardiac Arrhythmia Institute
St. David's Medical Center
Austin, TX, USA

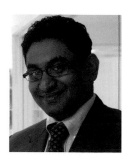

Prashanthan Sanders, MD
Centre for Heart Rhythm Disorders
Royal Adelaide Hospital
North Terrace, Adelaide, Australia

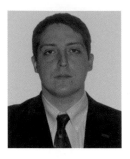

Pasquale Santangeli, MD
Texas Cardiac Arrhythmia Institute
St. David's Medical Center
Austin, TX, USA

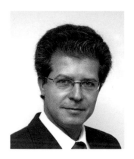

Vincenzo Santinelli, MD
Arrhythmology Department
Villa Maria Cecilia Hospital
Cotignola, Italy

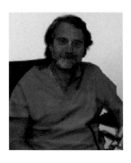

Mauricio Scanavacca, MD
Heart Institute
University of Sao Paulo Medical School
Sao Paulo, Brazil

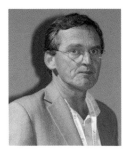

Martin J. Schalij, MD
Cardiology Department
Leiden Hospital
Leiden, The Netherlands

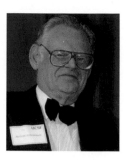

Melvin M. Scheinman, MD
Cardiac Electrophysiology Department
University of California
San Francisco, CA, USA

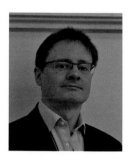

Richard J. Schilling, MD
Cardiology Department
St Bartholomew's Hospital
London, UK

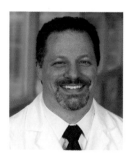

Robert A. Schweikert, MD
Cardiology Department
Akron General Medical Center
Akron, OH, USA

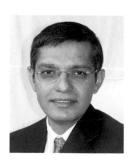

Dipen Shah, MD
Cardiology Cantonal Hospital of Geneva
Geneva, Switzerland

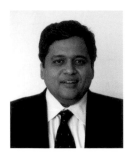

Kalyanam Shivkumar, MD
UCLA Cardiac Arrhythmia Center
David Geffen School of Medicine at UCLA
Los Angeles, CA, USA

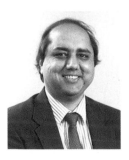

Jasbir Sra, MD
Aurora Cardiovascular Services
Aurora Sinai Medical Center
Milwaukee, WI, USA

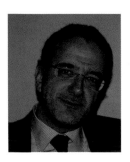

Sakis Themistoclakis, MD
Cardiovascular Department
Dell'Angelo Hospital
Mestre, Italy

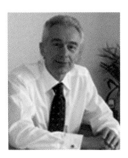

Claudio Tondo, MD
Arrhythmology Department
Centro Cardiologico Monzino
Milan, Italy

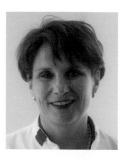

Isabelle C. van Gelder, MD
Cardiology Department
University Medical Center Groningen
Groningen, The Netherlands

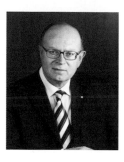

Panos E. Vardas, MD
Cardiology Department
Heraklion University Hospital
Heraklion, Greece

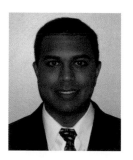

Atul Verma, MD
Cardiology Department
Southlake Regional Health Center
Toronto, ON, Canada

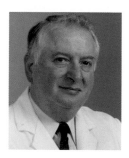

Albert L. Waldo, MD
Harrington-McLaughlin Heart & Vascular Institute
Division of Cardiovascular Medicine
University Hospitals Case Medical Center
Cleveland, OH, USA

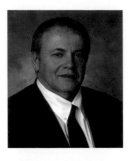

David J. Wilber, MD
Cardiology Department
Loyola University Medical Center
Chicago, IL, USA

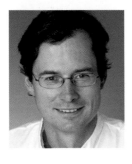

Stephan Willems, MD
Cardiology and Electrophysiology Department
Herzzentrum Hamburg GmbH University
Hamburg, Germany

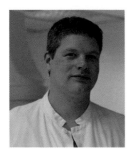

Erik Wissner, MD
Cardiology Department
Asklepios Klinik St. Georg
Hamburg, Germany

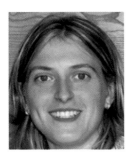

Francesca Zuffada, MD
Arrhythmology Department
Villa Maria Cecilia Hospital
Cotignola, Italy

VeniceChart task force composition

VeniceChart Task Force Co-Chairmen

Andrea Natale, MD, FACC, FESC, FHRS
Antonio Raviele, MD, FESC, FHRS

VeniceChart Task Force Working Groups

Anatomy of structures relevant to atrial fibrillation ablation
Siew Y. Ho, MD—*Working Group Chairman*
Cristina Basso, MD
José A. Cabrera, MD
Andrea Corrado, MD
Jeronimo Farré, MD
Josef Kautzner, MD
Roberto De Ponti, MD—*Working Group Liaison Member*

Pathophysiology of atrial fibrillation
José Jalife, MD—*Working Group Chairman*
Maurits Allessie, MD
Charles Antzelevitch, MD
Yoshito Iesaka, MD
Warren M. Jackman, MD
Melvin M. Scheinman, MD
Shih-Ann Chen, MD—*Working Group Liaison Member*

Techniques and technologies for atrial fibrillation catheter ablation
Karl H. Kuck, MD—*Working Group Chairman*
Pedro Adragao, MD
David J. Burkhardt, MD
Pierre Jaïs, MD
David Keane, MD
Hiroshi Nakagawa, MD
Robert A. Schweikert, MD
Jasbir Sra, MD
Vivek K. Reddy, MD—*Working Group Liaison Member*

Endpoints of catheter ablation for atrial fibrillation
Michel Haïssaguerre, MD—*Working Group Chairman*
Conor Barrett, MD
Luigi Di Biase, MD
Sabine Ernst, MD
Fiorenzo Gaita, MD
Javier E. Sanchez, MD
Prashanthan Sanders, MD
Richard J. Schilling, MD
Stephan Willems, MD—*Working Group Liaison Member*

Patient management pre-, during-, and postablation
David J. Wilber, MD—*Working Group Chairman*
Etienne Aliot, MD
Edward B. Gerstenfeld, MD
Chu-Pak Lau, MD
Martin J. Schalij, MD
Dipen Shah, MD
Hans Kottkamp, MD—*Working Group Liaison Member*

Periprocedural and long-term anticoagulation
Stuart J. Connolly, MD—*Working Group Chairman*
David Callans, MD
Mélèze Hocini, MD
Gregory Y.H. Lip, MD
Gregory F. Michaud, MD
Albert L. Waldo, MD
Sakis Themistoclakis, MD—*Working Group Liaison Member*

Periprocedural and late complications
Francis E. Marchlinski, MD—*Working Group Chairman*
Thomas Arentz, MD
Rodney P. Horton, MD
Hakan Oral, MD
Antonio Rossillo, MD
Eduardo Saad, MD
Mauricio Scanavacca, MD
Riccardo Cappato, MD—*Working Group Liaison Member*

Short- and long-term efficacy of catheter ablation procedures for atrial fibrillation
Hugh Calkins, MD—*Working Group Chairman*
Emanuele Bertaglia, MD
Antonio Berruezo, MD
Aldo Bonso, MD
Jonathan M. Kalman, MD
Moussa Mansour, MD
Atul Verma, MD—*Working Group Liaison Member*

Indications to atrial fibrillation ablation and cost-effectiveness
Eric N. Prystowsky, MD—*Working Group Chairman*
Josep Brugada, MD
Samuel Lévy, MD
Matthew Reynolds, MD
Vincenzo Santinelli, MD
Panos E. Vardas, MD
Francesca Zuffada, MD
Carlo Pappone, MD—*Working Group Liaison Member*

Clinical trials on atrial fibrillation/future perspectives
A. John Camm, MD—*Working Group Chairman*
Carina Blomström-Lundqvist, MD
Paul Dorian, MD
Stefan H. Hohnloser, MD
Carlos A. Morillo, MD
Pasquale Santangeli, MD
Isabelle C. van Gelder, MD
Erik Wissner, MD
Paulus Kirchhof, MD—*Working Group Liaison Member*

Surgical approach/ablation
Ralph Damiano Jr.—*Working Group Chairman*
Stefano Benussi, MD
Young-Hoon Kim, MD
Jos G. Maessen, MD
Helmut Mair, MD
Domenico Mangino, MD
Kalyanam Shivkumar, MD
James R. Edgerton—*Working Group Liaison Member*

Hospital equipment and facilities, personnel, training requirements, and competences

Douglas L. Packer, MD—*Working Group Chairman*
Johannes Brachmann, MD
Paolo Della Bella, MD
Luc J. Jordaens, MD
José L. Merino, MD
Claudio Tondo, MD
Gerhard Hindricks, MD—*Working Group Liaison Member*

List of abbreviations

2D	two-dimensional
3D	three-dimensional
7-d HM	7-day Holter monitoring
AA	antiarrhythmic
AADs	antiarrhythmic drugs
AATAC	*A*blation versus *A*miodarone for *T*reatment of *A*fib in patients with *C*HF
ACC	American College of Cardiology
ACGME	American Accreditation Council of Graduate Medical Education
ACT	activated clotting time
ADVICE	*AD*enosine following pulmonary *V*ein *I*solation to target dormant *C*onduction *E*limination
AF	atrial fibrillation
AF-CHF	atrial fibrillation and congestive heart failure
AFL	atrial flutter
AFNET	*A*trial *F*ibrillation competence *NET*work
AFSS	atrial fibrillation severity scale
AHA	American Heart Association
AMICA	*A*trial fibrillation *M*anagement *I*n *C*ongestive heart failure with *A*blation
APAF	*A*blation for *P*aroxysmal *A*trial *F*ibrillation
APD	action potential duration
ARC-HF	*A*blation versus medical *R*ate *C*ontrol for atrial fibrillation in patients with *H*eart *F*ailure
AVN	AV node
AVRT/AVNRT	atrioventricular reciprocating tachycardia/atrioventricular nodal reciprocating tachycardia
CABANA	*C*atheter *AB*lation versus *AN*tiarrhythmic drug therapy for *A*trial Fibrillation
CABG	coronary artery bypass grafting
CACAF	*C*atheter *A*blation for the *C*ure of *A*trial *F*ibrillation
CAF	chronic atrial fibrillation
CECC	conventional extra-corporeal circulation
CFAE	complex fractionated atrial electrogram
CFE	complex fractionated electrograms

CHADS	*C*ongestive heart failure *H*ypertension *A*ge *D*iabetes *S*troke
CHF	congestive heart failure
CMC	circular mapping catheter
CMP	Cox-maze procedure
CO	cross over
CPVA	circumferential pulmonary vein ablation
CS	coronary sinus
CT	computed tomography
CTE	crista terminalis
CV	cardiovascular
DC	direct current
DFs	dominant frequencies
EAM	electroanatomic mapping
EAST	*E*arly treatment of *A*trial fibrillation for *S*troke prevention *T*rial
ECG	electrocardiography
ECM	extracellular matrix
EGMs	electrograms
EHRA	European Heart Rhythm Association
ELR	external loop recorder
ESC	European Society of Cardiology
FAPs	fractionated atrial potentials
FFT	fast Fourier transform
GCV	great cardiac vein
GNs	ganglions
GP	ganglionated plexi
GWAS	genome-wide association studies
HCM	hypertrophic cardiomyopathy
HFS	high-frequency stimulation
HiFU	high-intensity frequency-focused ultrasound
HRS	high-rate stimulation
IAS	interatrial septum
ICD/CRT-D	implantable cardioverter defibrillator/cardiac resynchronization therapy + defibrillator
ICE	intracardiac echocardiography
ICER	incremental cost-effectiveness ratio
ICS	intercostal space
ICV	inferior caval vein
INHS	Italian National Health Service
INR	international normalized ratio
ITT	intention to treat
LA	left atrium
LAA	left atrial appendage

LAEF	LA ejection fraction
LARFA	left atrium radiofrequency ablation
LAT/FL	left atrial tachycardia/flutter
LI	left inferior
LIPV	left inferior pulmonary vein
LMWH	low molecular weight heparin
LPA	left pulmonary artery
LS	left superior
LSPV	left superior pulmonary vein
LVEF	left ventricular ejection fraction
LVF	left ventricular function
MCOT	mobile continuous outpatient telemetry
MECC	minimized extra-corporeal circulation
MLWHF	Minnesota living with heart failure
MMPs	matrix metalloproteinases
MPO	myeloperoxidase
MR	magnetic resonance
MRI	magnetic resonance imaging
MV	mitral valve
NA	not available
NR	not reported
NSR	normal sinus rhythm
OAC	oral anticoagulation
OS	orifice
PAF	paroxysmal atrial fibrillation
PFO	patent foramen ovale
PLA	posterior left atrium
PM	pacemaker
PN	phrenic nerve
PVAI	pulmonary vein antrum isolation
PVI	pulmonary vein isolation
PVs	pulmonary veins
QALY	quality-adjusted life year
QoL	quality of life
RA	right atrium
RAA	right atrial appendage
RAAFT	*Radiofrequency Ablation versus Antiarrhythmic drugs for atrial Fibrillation Treatment*
RAS	renin-angiotensin system
RF	radiofrequency
RFA	radiofrequency ablation
RFCA	radiofrequency catheter ablation
RI	right inferior
RIPV	right inferior pulmonary vein

RPA	right pulmonary artery
RS	right superior
RSPV	right superior pulmonary vein
SAN	sino-atrial node
SARA	*S*tudy of *A*blation versus antia*R*rhythmic drugs in persistent *A*trial fibrillation
SHD	structural heart disease
SNS	sympathetic nervous system
SVC	superior vena cava
SVCI	Superior vena cava isolation
TCL	tachycardia cycle length
TEE	transesophageal echocardiogram
TEs	thromboembolic events
TGF	transforming growth factor
TIA	transient ischemic attack
TSP	transseptal puncture
TTE	transthoracic echocardiography
TTEM	transtelephonic electrocardiographic monitoring
VASc	vascular disease age
VPSI	vasovagal pacemaker study
XLL	extra linear lesions in left atrium

CHAPTER 1

Anatomy of structures relevant to atrial fibrillation ablation

Siew Y. Ho[1], Cristina Basso[2], José A. Cabrera[3], Andrea Corrado[4], Jeronimo Farré[5], Josef Kautzner[6], Roberto De Ponti[7]

[1]Cardiac Morphology Department, Royal Brompton Hospital, Imperial College, London, UK
[2]Cardiovascular Pathology Department, University of Padua Medical School, Padua, Italy
[3]Arrhythmia Unit, Cardiology Department, Quirón Hospital, Universidad Europea de Madrid, Madrid, Spain
[4]Cardiology Department, Dell'Angelo Hospital, Venice-Mestre, Italy
[5]Cardiology Department, Jiménez Díaz-Capio Fundation, Madrid, Spain
[6]Cardiology Department, Institute for Clinical and Experimental Medicine, Prague, Czech Republic
[7]Cardiology Department, Circolo Hospital and Macchi Foundation, Varese, Italy

Introduction

Over the last few years, PVs have represented the cornerstone for catheter ablation of AF. Therefore, research has focused on their anatomy, histology, and peculiar electrophysiologic features. The data gathered from these studies have provided new insights in their morphologies and electrical function with a parallel improvement in patient care. However, as the ablation treatment of AF increases, the electrophysiologists' interest has moved also to other structures that are directly or indirectly involved in the AF ablation procedures. These structures may be of interest for the access to the LA (atrial septum/fossa ovalis), for their role as sources of atrial ectopic activities (SVC, LAA/ligament of Marshall), for their implications in the ablation strategy (mitral isthmus) or in interatrial conduction (accessory interatrial connection pathways), for their role in the pathophysiology of AF (GP), and for their possible involvement in severe complications (PNs and esophagus).

In this chapter, after describing the morphology of the LA and PVs, we focus on the above-mentioned anatomical structures, which have become of interest for the electrophysiologist in the perspective of AF ablation procedures.

Atrial Fibrillation Ablation, 2011 Update: The State of the Art based on the VeniceChart International Consensus Document, First Edition. Edited by Andrea Natale and Antonio Raviele.
© 2011 John Wiley & Sons, Ltd. Published 2011 by John Wiley & Sons, Ltd.

Left atrium

The LA has a venous component that receives the PVs, a finger-like atrial appendage, and shares the septum with the RA. The major part of the atrium, including the septal component, is relatively smooth-walled, whereas the appendage is rough with pectinate muscles (Figure 1.1). The smoothest parts are

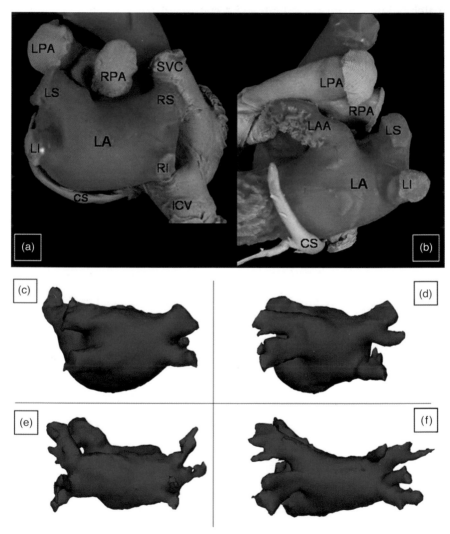

Figure 1.1 (a) The endocast viewed from the posterior aspect shows the proximity of the right PVs (RS and RI) to the atrial septum. Note also the RPA immediately above the roof of the LA. (b) The endocast viewed from the left shows the rough-walled LAA and its relationship to the LS. The CS passes inferior to the inferior wall of the LA. (c) to (e) are variations of PV arrangement from CT angio: (c) separate PVs on left side, (d) short common trunk on left side (the most common pattern), (e) long common trunk on left side (about 15%), and (f) supranumerary PVs on right side (about 20–25%).

the superior and posterior walls that make up the pulmonary venous component and the vestibule. Seemingly uniform, the walls are composed of one to three or more overlapping layers of differently aligned myocardial fibers, with marked regional variations in thickness [1] (Figure 1.2). The superior wall, or dome, is the thickest part of LA (3.5–6.5 mm), whereas the anterior wall just behind the proximal ascending aorta is usually the thinnest (1.5–4.8 mm) [2]. Also the posterior wall, especially between the superior PVs, is thin, approximately 2.5 mm in thickness. Normal LA end-systolic dimensions as measured

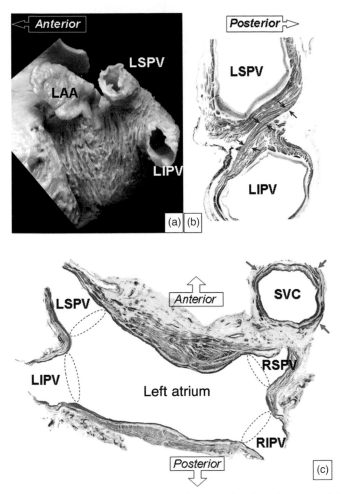

Figure 1.2 (a) The LA viewed from the left side and dissected to show the myocardial strands extending over the LSPV and LIPV. The LAA is finger-like in shape. (b) This histologic section taken through the left PVs shows myocardial strands crossing between the veins (blue arrows). Masson's trichrome stain. (c) This histologic section shows the four PVs with myocardial extensions (stained brown) over the outer surface of the veins. The ovals indicate the venoatrial junctions. Note the nonuniform thickness of the left atrial walls. The SVC is seen in cross section with its myocardial sleeve (green arrows). Elastic van Geison stain.

on cross-sectional echocardiography in the four-chamber view demonstrate the major axis to range from 4.1 to 6.1 cm (mean 5.1 cm) and from 2.3 to 3.5 cm/m^2 when indexed to body surface area. The minor axis ranges from 2.8 to 4.3 cm (mean 3.5 cm) and from 1.6 to 2.4 cm/m^2 when indexed.

Pulmonary veins

The presence of myocardial muscle extensions ("sleeves") covering the outside of PVs in mammals and in humans has been recognized for many years and are regarded as part of the mechanism regulating PV flow [3] (Figure 1.2). PVs are commonly identified as the source of rapid electrical activity triggering AF. This combines with the histological observation of P cells, transitional cells, and Purkinje cells in the myocardial sleeves of human PVs [4]. Interestingly, computerized high-density mapping demonstrated the possibility of proximal PV foci, triggering AF in humans [5]. Over the past several years, these anatomic and functional observations have conditioned a progressive change of the ablation strategy for PV electrical disconnection from the structural details of the distal PV branches to the anatomy of the venoatrial junction and from a segmental to a circumferential approach. Although PVI in the proximal venoatrial junction may be more challenging to achieve consistently due to its increased thickness as compared to less proximal areas, this strategy is expected not only to reduce the incidence of postablation PV stenosis but also to increase procedural efficacy.

Anatomic studies and studies using CT and MRI have reported the presence of significant anatomic variants of dimensions, shape, and branching of the PVs [6–10] (Figure 1.1). Typical anatomy with four distinct PV ostia is present in approximately 20–60% of subjects, while a very frequent anatomic variant is the presence of a short or long common left trunk, observed in up to 75–80% of the cases. The presence of supernumerary PVs, mainly right middle PVs or right upper PVs with a distinct os from the RSPV, is reported in 14–25% of the cases [11–13]. Intensive use of preprocedural 3D imaging with CT or MR scan in multiple centers has resulted in multiple reports of rare anatomic variants of PVs, such as the common os or trunk of the inferior PVs [14] and the posterior accessory PV [15]. The presence of one, two, or three PV variants in the same patient has been observed in 34%, 12%, and 2% of the cases, respectively [12].

There is general agreement that, albeit with a marked degree of interindividual variability, myocardial muscle fibers extend from the LA into all the PVs at a length of 1–3 cm; muscular sleeve is thickest at the proximal end of the veins (1–1.5 mm) and it then gradually tapers distally (Figure 1.2). Usually the sleeve is thickest at the inferior wall of the superior PVs and at the superior wall of the inferior PVs, although significant variations can be observed in individual cases. Frequently, muscular fibers are found circumferentially around the entire LA–PV junction but the muscular architecture is complex, with frequent segmental disconnections and abrupt changes in fiber orientation that may act as anatomical substrates for local reentry. Recently, an anatomical study [16] has highlighted some peculiar anatomical features of the interpulmonary isthmus, relevant for PVI by catheter ablation. This anatomic structure, which separates the ipsilateral PVs (the so-called carina), is the place where crossing fibers connecting the ipsilateral PVs are found, in a region where the myocardial PV sleeves may be in some cases as thick as 3.2 mm with intervenous muscular connections located epicardially, at a distance of 2.5 ± 0.5 mm for the left-sided PVs (Figure 1.2). In addition to the interpulmonary carinas, there is another notable "ridge"—the posterolateral ridge of the LA—that separates the orifice of the LAA from the orifices of the left PVs (see Section "Left atrial ridge and ligament of Marshall").

Atrial septum/fossa ovalis

Most of all, the anatomy of the atrial septum is of interest for the electrophysiologist for a safe transseptal catheterization. It is important to understand that the atrial septum does not correspond to the entire septal wall of the RA, as visualized by fluoroscopy. Instead, it is restricted to the fossa ovalis valve and the adjacent margin of its raised muscular rim (limbus) when seen from the right atrial aspect [17] (Figure 1.3). At particular risk of procedural complication is the anterior region of the limbus fossa ovalis, which is in close anatomical relationship with the aortic mound and is seen as a protuberance into the right atrial cavity. Puncture in this area is likely to allow the needle to enter the transverse pericardial sinus resulting in a high risk of aortic perforation.

The fossa ovalis may be either circular or oval, with approximately an average vertical diameter of 19 mm and an average horizontal diameter of 10 mm

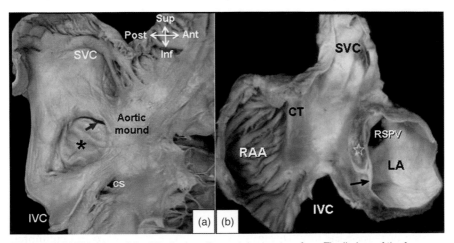

Figure 1.3 (a) This view of the RA displays the septal aspect *en face*. The limbus of the fossa ovalis surrounds a redundant and aneurismal-looking valve of the fossa (•). The blue arrows points to the slit-like PFO. (b) The atrial chambers cut in longitudinal section shows the infolding at the limbus (star) compared to the thin valve of the fossa (arrow).

Kyphoscoliosis
Straight back syndrome
Pectus excavatum
Obesity
Persistence of LS vena cava
Pericardial agenesia
Dextrocardia
Aortic or MV disease
Marked dilatation of the ascending aorta
Marked left ventricular hypertrophy

Table 1.1 Congenital or acquired diseases potentially affecting the location of the fossa ovalis.

[17], while its area varies from 1.5 to 3.4 cm^2 in adults [18–20]. The thin fossa is approximately 1–3 mm thick in normal hearts and has a bilaminar arrangement of myocytes with variable amounts of fibrous tissue [21]. Therefore, this is the target area where the TSP is expected to be easier. In the general patient population, the resistance of the fossa ovalis to puncture by the transseptal needle is not clearly predicted by its thickness, assessed by preprocedure transesophageal ecocardiography [22], nor by other clinical variables [23]. In patients undergoing multiple transseptal catheterization procedures, the fossa ovalis may become resistant to repeated punctures, possibly for a fibrotic reaction in the healing process after the first puncture. The location of the fossa ovalis varies from case to case. Table 1.1 lists abnormalities of the thorax or of the cardiovascular system that may result in displacement of the fossa ovalis. Since the limbus is an infolding of the right atrial wall with epicardial fat in between (Figure 1.3), it can become quite thick especially in its superior, posterior, and inferior margins. Indeed, in some patients, the epicardial fat may increase the thickness to 1–2 cm in the normal heart. TSP through the limbus is less likely to be satisfactory since the tissue thickness can hinder needle penetration or maneuverability of the transseptal sheath after puncture. Furthermore, septal thickness of >2 cm on noninvasive imaging is increasingly reported as indicative of lipomatous hypertrophy, with incidence up to 8% on echocardiography. On cross-sectional imaging, the septum appears like a "dumb-bell" [24] encroaching upon access to the thin fossa, which is not affected by fat deposition, especially in cases with small fossa area.

Aneurysmal fossa or so-called septal aneurysm has an incidence of 0.2–1.9% in echocardiographic reports. It is detected as a saccular excursion of >1 cm of the fossa membrane away from the plane of the atrial septum. Approximately a third is associated with a PFO. Often, the fossa membrane is thinner, devoid of muscle cells and mainly composed of connective tissue. PFO existing with or without aneurismal fossa is common, occurring in 10–35% of the population. It represents a lack of adhesion of the antero-cephalad border of the membrane to the limbus (Figure 1.3). If this portal is to be used for septal crossing, it is important to note its size and distance to the antero-cephalad wall of the LA to prevent accidental exit from the heart and to ensure adequate maneuverability for reaching the target areas in the LA.

Superior vena cava

There is a great bulk of evidence that AF is triggered mainly from ectopic foci originating from the PVs and that PVI is a key step in catheter ablation of this arrhythmia [25]. However, ectopic beats initiating AF may occasionally arise from non-PV foci, such as the SVC, left atrial posterior free wall, ligament of Marshall, crista terminalis, and/or CS. On the basis of previous studies, the SVC houses the majority of non-PV foci [26–28].

Anatomically, atrial myocardium extends into the SVC (Figure 1.4) much like what occurs at the CS and around the PV [29,30] (Figure 1.2). Such myocardial extensions into both caval veins were found in the majority of human beings (76% of cases), both with and without a history of AF. Their average length in the SVC reached 13.7 ± 13.9 mm (maximum, up to 47 mm) and in the inferior vena cava, 14.6 ± 16.7 mm (maximum, up to 61 mm). The thickness of atrial myocardium extending into the CVs was 1.2 ± 1.0 mm (maximum, 4 mm) for the SVC and 1.2 ± 0.9 mm for the inferior vena cava (maximum, 3 mm).

Several groups studied incremental value of SVC isolation in addition to PVI in patients with paroxysmal or persistent AF [31–32]. The Cleveland Clinic group revealed SVC triggers in 12% of 190 patients, and isolation of the SVC prevented recurrences of AF [31]. In Mestre [32], a total of 320 consecutive patients who had been referred to for a first attempt of AF ablation

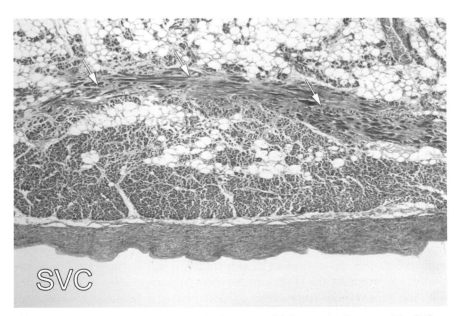

Figure 1.4 An example of photomicrograph of a myocardial sleeve extending around the SVC. The sleeve is located next to the adventitia of the caval vein. Its fibers are mainly circular and peripherally intermingled with fat cells. Longitudinally oriented fibers (arrows) are partially fibrotic.

were randomized into two groups—PVI only and PVI with SVC isolation. SVC isolation was performed on 134 of the 160 patients (84%), and could not be accomplished in the remaining 26 patients because of PN proximity or due the lack of local potentials. Comparison of the outcome data between the two groups, after a follow-up of 12 months, revealed a significant difference in total procedural success solely with patients manifesting paroxysmal AF (56/73 [77%] Group I vs. 55/61 [90%] Group II; $p = .04$; OR 2.78). On the other hand, a Chinese group [33] studied 106 cases (58 males, average age 66.0 + 8.8 years) with paroxysmal AF who were allocated randomly to two groups: PVI only ($n = 54$) and PVI with SVCI ($n = 52$). No difference in outcome was revealed during a mean follow-up of $4 + 2$ months. Therefore, the evidence that SVC isolation in addition to PVI reduces the recurrence of AF is not overwhelming.

For the above reasons, the indications for SVC isolation should be decided upon carefully because SVC isolation may cause some complications such as PN and/or sinus node injury. According to a study by Higuchi et al. [34], SVC sleeve length ≥30 mm and maximum amplitude of SVC potential ≥1.0 mV strongly predicted an SVC focus of AF (100% sensitivity, 94% specificity).

Technically, SVC isolation is most frequently performed using the CMC above the junction between the RA and SVC [31,35–37]. ICE proved a useful strategy to perform ablation at the level of the lower border of the RPA in order to avoid ablation close the sinus node. Pacing from ablation catheter with a high output is used to minimize PN injury. The rate of reconduction seems to be lower than after PVI [37].

Left atrial appendage

In a review of published papers, it was reported that in approximately 90% of patients with nonrheumatic AF thrombi were located in the LAA, making this finger-like extension of the LA of great strategic importance for stroke prophylaxis [38]. It is also a source of focal atrial tachycardia after ablation of long-lasting persistent AF [39]. Recent investigations have demonstrated extra-PV atrial foci after PVI originating from the appendage and that the junctional area between the left appendage [40] and the LA body is important in the AF process acting as a source of activity spreading to the rest of the atrium [41]. Although generally long and narrow in appearance, the external aspect of the finger shows multiple crenellations giving wide variations in number and arrangement of lobes (Figure 1.2a). Internally, the endocardial aspect is lined with muscle bundles of varied thicknesses akin to the pectinate muscles of the RA, but they are arranged in whorl-like fashion instead of in an array since there is no equivalent of a crista terminalis in the LA. In between the muscle bundles, the wall is paper-thin. The appendage communicates with the atrial chamber through an oval-shaped os. In some hearts, the atrial wall around the os can also be thin [42] (Figure 1.5). A study of postmortem and explanted hearts revealed the atrial appendage from patients with AF to

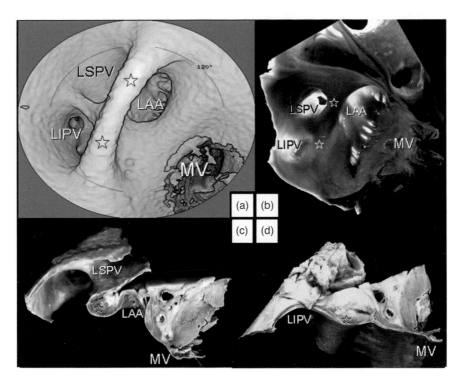

Figure 1.5 (a) This 3D rendering of a CT scan shows the endocardial surface of the LA with a pronounced "ridge" (stars) bordering the anterior margin of the left pulmonary venous orifices. (b) The left atrial ridge (stars) displayed in similar fashion as the image shown in (a). Transillumination reveals the thin areas of the walls, especially in the LAA. (c) This cut through the LSPV, the LAA, and the muscular ridge (star) shows its rounded profile and enclosing epicardial fatty tissues. (d) This cut through the LIPV shows a flatter ridge (star).

have three times the volume of those in sinus rhythm [43]. Furthermore, the endocardial surface was smoother and associated with more extensive endocardial fibroelastosis in those with AF. These features could contribute to appendage dysfunction and predisposition to thrombus formation [43].

Left atrial ridge and ligament of Marshall

A certain degree of variability is observed in the posterolateral ridge that is integral to the left PVI line (Figure 1.5). On the endocardial surface, it appears like a ridge but is actually an infolding of the left atrial wall separating the left PVs from the atrial appendage. On the epicardial aspect of the infolding runs, the remnant of the vein of Marshall covered over by fatty tissues containing abundant autonomic nerve bundles and ganglia [44] (Figure 1.5). In approximately 66% of hearts, the fold also contains a branch from the circumflex artery that supplies the left lateral wall that, in a smaller proportion, continues to supply the sinus node [45,46].

The muscular wall of the ridge contains extensions of the leftward branches of Bachmann's bundle. Measurements made on 32 cadaver heart specimens showed the ridge to be narrower at its superior border with the LSPV orifice compared to its inferior border with the inferior PV orifice (range 2.2–6.3 mm vs. 6.2–12.3 mm). Moreover, the endocardial aspect of this ridge may be flat, round, or pointed in profile. The first shape may be more favorable for catheter stability when positioned in this area for ablation, whereas the second and third could be very unfavorable. Overall, the ridge was <5 mm wide in 75% of hearts, suggesting that achieving catheter stability for adequate contact can be challenging in most cases [9,45].

Mitral isthmus

Linear ablation between the inferior border of the orifice of the LIPV and the mitral annulus is carried out in AF ablation to prevent recurrences. This line, dubbed the mitral isthmus, crosses the atrial vestibule, which comprises the inferior left atrial wall measuring 2–5 cm long (Figure 1.6). On its epicardial aspect runs the GCV as the vessel approaches the CS. The wall of the isthmus ranges from 2 to 8 mm in myocardial thickness. Its endocardial surface may contain pits and troughs where the atrial wall becomes exceptionally thin [47].

Interatrial conduction pathways alternative to Bachmann's bundle

In normal hearts, the sinus impulse is quickly propagated to the anterior wall of the LA over the Bachmann's bundle, which functionally represents the prevalent interatrial conduction pathway [48]. When a conduction delay or block occurs over the Bachmann's bundle or when an atrial arrhythmia or a paced rhythm from a site different from the high RA are present, accessory interatrial connections may become predominant and play a major role in the right-to-left or left-to-right atrial propagation. Moreover, delayed conduction over the Bachmann's bundle associated with interatrial conduction occurring over alternative interatrial pathways is peculiarly observed in patients with AF [49]. These accessory interatrial connections might be multiple in the same patient, show an epicardial course in direct contact with epicardial fat, and be accompanied by numerous neural fibers and ganglia [19]. They cross the interatrial groove posteriorly, at the level of the antrum of the superior and inferior PVs, or inferiorly, at the level of the inferomedial LA and CS, which exhibits myocardial sleeves surrounding its proximal tract [2,19,48] (Figure 1.6 (b1)). Finally, also fascicles located at the level of the fossa ovalis or at the level of the CS os may serve as accessory interatrial pathways [19]. Ablation in the medial region of the LA, along the septum and/or the proximal CS,

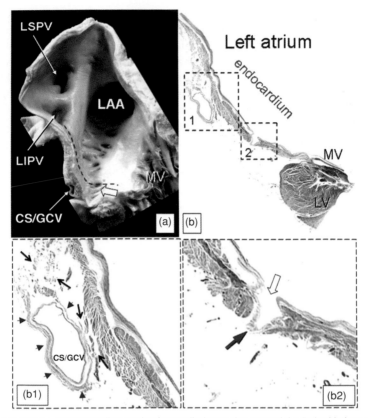

Figure 1.6 (a) The red broken line marks the vestibular portion termed the "mitral isthmus." It lies between the inferior margin of the LIPV and the annulus of the MV. Its endocardial surface may contain pits and furrows (open arrow), while its epicardial surface is traversed by the CS or its continuity with the GCV. (b) This histologic section of a mitral isthmus shows the fibrous endocardial lining (stained green). Boxes 1 and 2 are enlarged: (b1) shows the CS/GCV with its own muscular sleeve (blue arrow heads) and muscular continuity with the left atrial wall (black arrows); (b2) shows a pit (open arrow) in the isthmus that entraps a catheter tip. Note the thinness of the wall at the bottom of the pit (red arrow). Masson's trichrome stain.

causing disruption of accessory interatrial connections and tissue debulking [50], may considerably alter the interatrial propagation during postablation organized atrial arrhythmias with unexpected modification of the surface P-wave morphology. This may occur even during typical isthmus-dependent AFL and leads to misdiagnosis of this arrhythmia [51].

Ganglionated plexi

The intrinsic cardiac nervous system influences cardiac rate, atrial and ventricular refractoriness, coronary blood flow, valve function, and atrial natriuretic peptide secretion, and it appears involved in many human heart disorders [52–54]. In particular, in paroxysmal AF although most investigations have focused on specific histological and electrophysiological properties of PVs, there are studies suggesting that some of the rapid PV firings can be induced and eliminated by stimulation and interruption of the intrinsic cardiac autonomic nervous system [55]. There is also clinical evidence that ablation of the main GP on the atria increases the success of the standard PVI by catheter ablation for AF. In other words, the active role of PVs in AF results from the high density of adrenergic and cholinergic nerves around PVs. The areas most suitable for autonomic nervous system modification procedures are located in the immediate vicinity of the PV-left atrial junction.

The topography and structure of the human epicardiac neural plexus has been carefully investigated by Pauza et al. [53,54]. It consists of a system of seven GPs that are epicardiac extensions of mediastinal nerves entering the heart through discrete sites of the so-called heart hilum. They are mostly concentrated at the fat pads and proceed separately into regions of innervation by seven pathways, on the courses of which epicardiac ganglia, as wide ganglionated fields, are located. From the arterial part of the heart hilum (i.e., around the ascending aorta and pulmonary trunk) nerves extend predominantly into the ventricles, while from the venous part of the heart hilum (i.e., around PVs and venae cavae) (Figures 1.7 and 1.8) intrinsic nerves go to both the atria and ventricles.

In general, the human RA is innervated by two subplexuses, the LA by three, the right ventricle by one, and the left ventricle by three subplexuses. The subplexuses have been named according to their topography and/or area in which subplexal post-GNs were extended: left coronary and right coronary (between the aorta and pulmonary trunk); ventral right atrial (at the superior interatrial sulcus and nonregularly on the ventral surface of the root of SVC); ventral left atrial (between the superior interatrial sulcus and left atrial nerve fold); left dorsal (at the left atrial nerve fold); middle dorsal (between the right and LSPVs and, nonregularly, between the both right PVs and inferior vena cava), and dorsal right atrial (between the SVC and RSPV). The structural organization of ganglia and nerves within subplexuses varies considerably from heart to heart and in relation to age.

The highest density of epicardiac ganglia was identified near the heart hilum, especially on the dorsal and dorsolateral surfaces of the LA, where up to 50% of all cardiac ganglia were located. In the study by Pauza et al. [54], the number of epicardiac ganglia identified for the human hearts ranged from 706 to 1560. The human heart contains on average 836 ± 76 epicardiac ganglia. The number of neurons identified for any epicardiac ganglion was significantly fewer in aged human compared with infants. By estimating the number of neurons within epicardiac ganglia and relating this to the number of ganglia in the human epicardium, it was calculated that approximately 43,000 intrinsic neurons might be present in the epicardiac neural plexus in adult hearts.

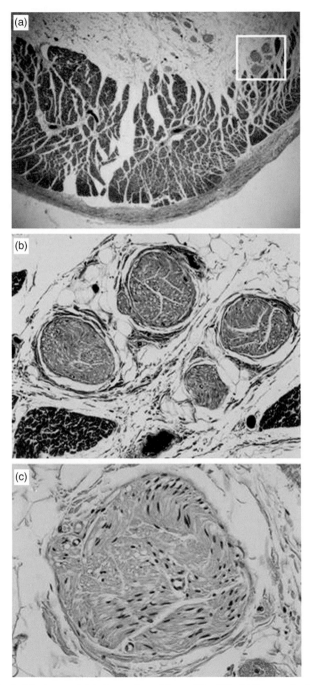

Figure 1.7 Roof of the human LA between the orifices of the PVs. (a) Panoramic view of the left atrial wall, consisting of epicardiac fat pad, myocardium, and thin endocardium. Trichrome azan stain. (b) Close-up of the boxed area in (a): at higher magnification, epicardiac ganglia are visible. (c) Normal epicardiac ganglion. Hematoxylin–eosin stain.

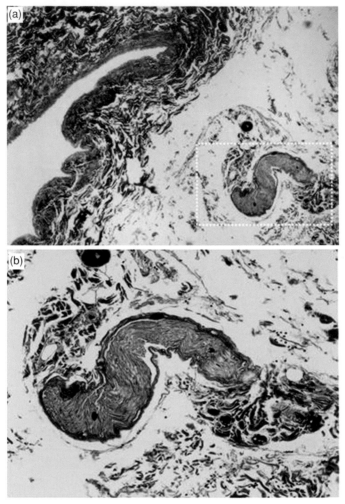

Figure 1.8 Histology of the left atrial wall close to the LIPV ostium. (a) A nerve is visible close to the LIPVs ostium (trichrome azan). (b) Close-up of the nerve fibers.

Phrenic nerves

The PNs and their accompanying pericardiophrenic artery and vein descend bilaterally adherent to the surface of the fibrous pericardium. The course of the right PN is in close proximity to the superior caval vein and the superior right PV. It is particularly close to the PV with a mean minimal distance of $2.1 + 0.4$ mm in a study made on cadavers. The same study found that the distance was <2 mm in a third of the cadavers, suggesting that it could be at risk of damage during right PV isolation [56]. The left PN takes an anterior (18%), lateral (59%), or posteroinferior (23%) course on the fibrous pericardium overlying the left heart. The lateral course passes over the tip of the LAA, while the posteroinferior course passes over the roof of the appendage os [57].

Esophagus

The close relationship of the esophagus to the LA exposes it to risk of inadvertent damage when ablative lesions are made in the posterior and inferior walls (Figure 1.9). It descends in a variable course, in midline or more toward the right or the left PVs and it has peristaltic movements. It is separated from the epicardial surface of the LA by the fibrous pericardium and a plane of fibrofatty tissues that contains the arterial supply to the esophagus as well as the vagus neural plexus. The distance between the endocardial surface of the LA and the esophageal wall was <5 mm in 40% of the specimens in a study performed on cadavers [58]. Taking into account the thickness of the left atrial wall, deep and large lesions can inflict injury to the esophageal arteries and vagal nerves even though the esophageal wall itself is not directly affected.

Measurements of the thickness of the posterior left atrial wall at levels corresponding to the midline in between the superior PVs, between the inferior PVs, and centrally showed the thinnest wall at the superior location [59]. Moreover, the wall at the inferior and central locations was significantly thinner in hearts from patients with AF compared to without AF (2.5 ± 1.3 mm vs. 2.9 ± 1.3 mm and 2.2 ± 1 mm vs. 2.6 ± 1 mm, respectively) [59].

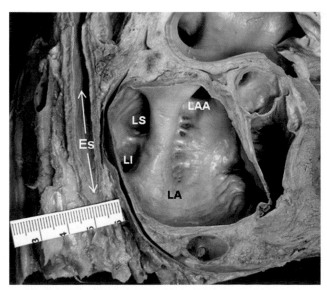

Figure 1.9 This sagittal section through the LA of a cadaver shows the proximity of the esophagus to the posterior wall of the LA. Note the nonuniform thickness of the LA wall, particularly at the level of the superior PV. (Picture courtesy of Professor Damian Sanchez-Quintana, University of Extremadura, Badajoz, Spain.)

Conclusions

Until the substrates for AF are fully clarified, atrial ablation procedures remain anatomically orientated. For improvements in efficacy and safety of the procedures, a comprehensive understanding of cardiac anatomy and the relationship of cardiac structures to neighboring structures is the first step. This chapter has reviewed the LA with particular emphasis on the atrial septum and highlighted cardiac and adjacent structures relevant to AF ablation.

References

1. Ho SY, Anderson RH, Sanchez-Quintana D. Atrial structure and fibres: Morphological basis of atrial conduction. Cardiovasc Res 2002; 54:325–336.
2. Ho SY, Sanchez-Quintana D, Cabrera JA, Anderson RH. Anatomy of the left atrium: Implications for radiofrequency ablation of atrial fibrillation. J Cardiovasc Electrophysiol 1999; 10:1525–1533.
3. Ho SY, Cabrera JA, Tran VH, Farré J, Anderson RH, Sanchez-Quintana D. Architecture of the pulmonary veins: Relevance to radiofrequency ablation. Heart 2001; 86:265–270.
4. Perez-Lugones A, McMahon JT, Ratliff NB, et al. Evidence of specialized conduction cells in human pulmonary veins of patients with atrial fibrillation. J Cardiovasc Electrophysiol 2003; 14:803–809.
5. De Ponti R, Tritto M, Lanzotti M, et al. Computerized high-density mapping of the pulmonary veins: new insights into their electrical activation in patients with atrial fibrillation. Europace 2004; 6:97–108.
6. Kato R, Lickfett L, Meininger G, Dickfeld T, Wu R, Juang G, Angkeow P, LaCorte J, Bluemke D, Berger R, Halperin H, Calkins H. Pulmonary vein anatomy in patients undergoing catheter ablation of atrial fibrillation: Lessons learned by use of magnetic resonance imaging. Circulation 2003; 107:2004–2010.
7. Scharf C, Sneider M, Case I, et al. Anatomy of the pulmonary veins in patients with atrial fibrillation and effects of segmental ostial ablation analyzed by computed tomography. J Cardiovasc Electrophysiol 2003; 14:150–155.
8. Ho SY, Cabrera JA, Sanchez-Quintana D. Anatomy of the pulmonary vein-atrium junction. In: Chen SA, Haissaguerre M, Zipes DP, eds. Thoracic Vein Arrhythmias. Mechanisms and Treatment. Blackwell Futura: Oxford; 2004, pp. 42–53.
9. Mansour M, Refaat M, Heist EK, Mela T, Cury R, Holmvang G, Ruskin J. Three-dimensional anatomy of the left atrium by magnetic resonance angiography: Implication for catheter ablation for atrial fibrillation. J Cardiovac Electrophysiol 2006; 17:719–723.
10. Mlcochova H, Tintera J, Porod V, Peichi O, Cihak R, Kautzner J. Magnetic resonance angiography of pulmonary veins: implications for catheter ablation of atrial fibrillation. Pacing Clin Electrophysiol 2005; 28:1073–1080.
11. De Ponti R, Marazzi R, Lumia D, Picciolo G, Biddau R, Fugazzola C, Salerno-Uriarte JA. Role of three-dimensional imaging integration in atrial fibrillation ablation. World J Cardiol 2010; 2:215–222.
12. Hamdan A, Charalampos K, Roettgen R, et al. Magnetic resonance imaging versus computed tomography for characterization of pulmonary vein morphology before radiofrequency catheter ablation of atrial fibrillation. Am J Cardiol 2009; 104:1540–1546.
13. Anselmino M, Blandino A, Beninati S, et al. Morphologic analysis of left atrial anatomy by magnetic resonance angiography in patients with atrial fibrillation: a large single center experience. J Cardiovasc Electrophysiol 2011; 22:1–7.

14. Marazzi R, De Ponti R, Lumia D, Fugazzola C, Salerno-Uriarte JA. Common trunk of the inferior pulmonary veins: an unexpected anatomical variant detected before ablation by multi-slice computed tomography. Europace 2007; 9:121.

15. Diaz-Caraballo E, Merino JL, Guzman G. Posterior accessory pulmonary veins and atrial fibrillation. Rev Esp Cardiol 2010; 63:224.

16. Cabrera JA, Ho, SY, Climent V, et al. Morphological evidence of muscular connections between contiguous pulmonary venous orifices: relevance of the interpulmonary isthmus for catheter ablation in atrial fibrillation. Heart Rhythm 2009; 6:1192–1198.

17. Tzeis S, Andrikopoulos G, Deisenhofer I, Ho SY, Theodorakis G. Transseptal catheterization: Considerations and caveats. Pacing Ciin Electrophysiol 2010; 33:231–242.

18. Shirani J, Zafari AM, Roberts WC. Morphologic features of fossa ovalis membrane aneurysm in the adult and its clinical significance. J Am Coll Cardiol 1995; 26:466–471.

19. Platonov PG, Mitrofanova L, Ivanov V, Ho SY. Substrates for intra-atrial and interatrial conduction in the atrial septum: Anatomical study on 84 human hearts. Heart Rhythm 2008; 5:1189–1195.

20. Babaliaros VC, Green JT, Lerakis S, Lloyd M, Block PC. Emerging application for transseptal left heart catheterization: old techniques for new procedures. J Am Coll Cardiol 2008; 51:2116–2122.

21. Ho SY, McCarthy KP. Anatomy of the left atrium for interventional electrophysiologists. Pacing Clin Electrophysiol 2010; 33:620–627.

22. Knecht S, Jais P, Nault I, et al. Radiofrequency puncture of the fossa ovalis for resistant transseptal access. Circ Arrhythmia Electrophysiol 2008; 1:169–174.

23. De Ponti R, Marazzi R, Picciolo G, Salerno-Uriarte JA. Use of a novel sharp-tip J-shaped guidewire to facilitate transseptal catheterization. Europace 2010; 12:668–673.

24. Fyke FE 3rd, Tajik AJ, Edwards WD, Seward JB. Diagnosis of lipomatous hypertrophy of the atrial septum by two-dimensional echocardiography. J Am Coll Cardiol 1983; 1:1352–1357.

25. Calkins H, Brugada J, Packer DL, Cappato R, Chen SA, Crijns HJ, Damiano RJ Jr, Davies DW, Haines DE, Haissaguerre M, Iesaka Y, Jackman W, Jais P, Kottkamp H, Kuck KH, Lindsay BD, Marchlinski FE, McCarthy PM, Mont JL, Morady F, Nademanee K, Natale A, Pappone C, Prystowsky E, Raviele A, Ruskin JN, Shemin RJ. Heart Rhythm Society; European Heart Rhythm Association; European Cardiac Arrhythmia Society; American College of Cardiology; American Heart Association; Society of Thoracic Surgeons. HRS/EHRA/ECAS expert consensus statement on catheter and surgical ablation of atrial fibrillation: Recommendations for personnel, policy, procedures and follow-up. A report of the Heart Rhythm Society (HRS) Task Force on Catheter and Surgical Ablation of Atrial Fibrillation developed in partnership with the European Heart Rhythm Association (EHRA) and the European Cardiac Arrhythmia Society (ECAS); in collaboration with the American College of Cardiology (ACC), American Heart Association (AHA), and the Society of Thoracic Surgeons (STS). Endorsed and approved by the governing bodies of the American College of Cardiology, the American Heart Association, the European Cardiac Arrhythmia Society, the European Heart Rhythm Association, the Society of Thoracic Surgeons, and the Heart Rhythm Society. Europace 2007; 9: 335–379.

26. Tsai CF, Tai CT, Hsieh MH, et al. Initiation of atrial fibrillation by ectopic beats originating from the superior vena cava: Electrophysiological characteristics and results of radiofrequency ablation. Circulation 2000; 102:67.

27. Shah D, Haissaguerre M, Jais P, Hocini M. Nonpulmonary vein foci: do they exist? Pacing Clin Electrophysiol 2003; 26:1631.

28. Lin WS, Tai CT, Hsieh MH, Tsai CF, Lin YK, Tsao HM, Huang JL, Yu WC, Yang SP, Ding YA, Chang MS, Chen SA. Catheter ablation of paroxysmal atrial fibrillation initiated by non-pulmonary vein ectopy. Circulation 2003; 107:3176–3183.

29. Asirvatham S, Friedman P, Packer D, Edwards W. Does atrial myocardium extend into the superior vena cava and azygous vein? Circulation 2001; 104:730.

30. Kholova I, Kautzner J. Morphology of atrial myocardial extensions into human caval veins: a postmortem study in patients with and without atrial fibrillation. Circulation 2004; 110:483–488.

31. Arruda M, Mlcochova H, Prasad SK, et al. Electrical Isolation of the Superior Vena Cava: An Adjunctive Strategy to Pulmonary Vein Antrum Isolation Improving the Outcome of AF Ablation. J Cardiovasc Electrophysiol 2007; 18:1261–1266.

32. Corrado A, Bonso A, Madalosso M, et al. Impact of systematic isolation of superior vena cava in addition to pulmonary vein antrum isolation on the outcome of paroxysmal, persistent, and permanent atrial fibrillation ablation: results from a randomized study. J Cardiovasc Electrophysiol 2010; 21:1–5.

33. Wang XH, Liu X, Sun Y-M, et al. Pulmonary vein isolation combined with superior vena cava isolation for atrial fibrillation ablation: a prospective randomized study. Europace 2008; 10:600–605.

34. Higuchi K, Yamauchi Y, Hirao K, et al. Superior vena cava as initiator of atrial fibrillation: factors related to its arrhythmogenicity. Heart Rhythm 2010; 7:1186–1191.

35. Macedo PG, Kapa S, Mears JA, Fratianni A, Asirvatham S. Correlative Anatomy for the Electrophysiologist: Ablation for Atrial Fibrillation. Part I: Pulmonary Vein Ostia, Superior Vena Cava, Vein of Marshall. J Cardiovasc Electrophysiol 2010; 21:721–730.

36. Goya M, Ouyang F, Ernst S, Volkmer M, Antz M, Kuck KH: Electroanatomic mapping and catheter ablation of breakthroughs from the right atrium to the superior vena cava in patients with atrial fibrillation. Circulation 2002; 106:1317–1320.

37. Muto M, Yamada T, Murakami Y, et al. Electrophysiologic characteristics and outcome of segmental ostial superior vena cava isolation in patients with paroxysmal atrial fibrillation initiated by superior vena cava ectopy: comparison with pulmonary vein isolation. J Electrocardiol 2007; 40:319–325.

38. Blackshear JL, Odell JA. Obliteration of the left atrial appendage to reduce stroke in cardiac surgical patients with atrial fibrillation. Ann Thorac Surg 1996; 61:755–759.

39. Takahashi Y, Takahashi A, Miyazaki S, et al. Electrophysiological characteristics of localized reentrant atrial tachycardia occurring after catheter ablation of long-lasting persistent atrial fibrillation. J Cardiovasc Electrophysiol 2009; 20:623–629.

40. Di Biase L, Burkhardt JD, Mohanty P, Sanchez J, Mohanty S, Horton R, Gallinghouse GJ, Bailey SM, Zagrodzky JD, Santangeli P, Hao S, Hongo R, Beheiry S, Themistoclakis S, Bonso A, Rossillo A, Corrado A, Raviele A, Al-Ahmad A, Wang P, Cummings JE, Schweikert RA, Pelargonio G, Dello Russo A, Casella M, Santarelli P, Lewis WR, Natale A. Left atrial appendage: an underrecognized trigger site of atrial fibrillation Circulation. 2010; 122:109–18.

41. Takahashi Y, Sanders P, Rotter M, Haissaguerre M. Disconnection of the left atrial appendage for elimination of foci maintaining atrial fibrillation. J Cardiovasc Electrophysiol 2005; 16:917–919.

42. Su P, McCarthy KP, Ho SY. Occluding the left atrial appendage: anatomical considerations. Heart 2008; 94:1166–1170.

43. Shirani J, Alaeddin J. Structural remodelling of the left atrial appendage in patients with chronic non-valvular atrial fibrillation: implications for thrombus formation, systemic

embolism, and assessment by transesophageal echocardiography. Cardiovasc Pathol 2000; 9:95–101.

44. Kim DT, Lai AC, Hwang C, et al. The ligament of Marshall: a structural analysis in human hearts with implications for atrial arrhythmias. J Am Coll Cardiol 2000; 36:1324–1327.

45. Cabrera JA, Ho SY, Climent V, Sanchez-Quintana. The architecture of the left lateral atrial wall: A particular anatomic region with implications for ablation of atrial fibrillation. Eur Heart J 2008; 29:356–362.

46. Busquet J, Fontan F, Anderson RH, Ho SY, Davies MJ. The surgical significance of the atrial branches of the coronary arteries. Int J Cardiol 1984; 6:223–234.

47. Wittkampf FHM, van Oosterhout MF, Loh P, et al. Where to draw the mitral isthmus line in catheter ablation of atrial fibrillation: histological analysis. Eur Heart J 2005; 26:689–695.

48. De Ponti R, Ho SY, Salerno-Uriarte JA, Tritto M, Spadacini G. Electroanatomic analysis of sinus impulse propagation in normal human atrial. J Cardiovasc Electrohysiol 2002; 13:1–10.

49. Jurkko R, Mantynen V, Letho M, Tapanainen JM, Montonen J, Parikka H, Toivonen L. Interatrial conduction in patients with paroxysmal atrial fibrillation and in healthy subjects. Int J Cardiol 2010; 145:455–460.

50. Udyavar AR, Huang SH, Chang SL, et al. Acute effect of circumferential pulmonary vein isolation on left atrial substrate. J Cardiovasc Electrophysiol 2009; 20:715–722.

51. Chugh A, Latchamsetty R, Oral H, Elmouchi D, Tschopp D, Reich S, Igic P, Lemerand T, Good E, Bogun F, Pelosi F, Morady F. Characteristics of cavotricuspid isthmus-dependent atrial flutter after left atrial ablation of atrial fibrillation. Circulation 2006; 113:609–615.

52. Armour JA, Murphy DA, Yuan BX, Macdonald S, Hopkins DA. Gross and microscopic anatomy of the human intrinsic cardiac nervous system. Anat Rec 1997; 247:289–298.

53. Pauza DH, Skripka V, Pauziene N, Stropus R. Anatomical study of the neural ganglionated plexus in the canine right atrium: implications for selective denervation and electrophysiology of the sinoatrial node in dog. Anat Rec 1999; 255:271–294.

54. Pauza DH, Skripka V, Pauziene N, Stropus R. Morphology, distribution, and variability of the epicardiac neural ganglionated subplexuses in the human heart. Anat Rec 2000; 259:353–382.

55. Scherlag BJ, Po S. The intrinsic cardiac nervous system and atrial fibrillation. Curr Opin Cardiol 2006; 21:51–54.

56. Sanchez-Quintana, Cabrera JA, Climent V, Farre J, Weiglein A, Ho SY. How close are the phrenic nerves to cardiac structures? Implications for cardiac interventionalists. J Cardiovasc Electrophysiol 2005; 16:309–313.

57. Sánchez-Quintana D, Ho SY, Climent V, Murillo M, Cabrera JA. Anatomic evaluation of the left phrenic nerve relevant to epicardial and endocardial catheter ablation: implications for phrenic nerve injury. Heart Rhythm 2009; 6:764–768.

58. Sánchez-Quintana D, Cabrera JA, Climent V, Farré J, de Mendonça MC, Ho SY. Anatomic relations between the esophagus and left atrium and relevance for ablation of atrial fibrillation. Circulation 2005; 112:1400–1405.

59. Platonov PG, Ivanov V, Ho SY, Mitrofanova L. Left atrial posterior wall thickness in patients with and without atrial fibrillation: Data from 298 consecutive autopsies. J Cardiovasc Electrophysiol 2008; 19:689–692.

CHAPTER 2

Pathophysiology of atrial fibrillation

**José Jalife[1], Maurits Allessie[2], Charles Antzelevitch[3],
Yoshito Iesaka[1], Warren M. Jackman[5], Melvin M. Scheinman[6],
Shih-Ann Chen[7]**

[1]University of Michigan, Ann Arbor, MI, USA
[2]Cardiovascular Research Institute Maastricht, Maastricht, The Netherlands
[3]Masonic Medical Research Laboratory Utica, NY, USA
[4]Tsuchiura Kyodo Hospital, Tsuchiura City, Japan
[5]Heart Rhythm Institute, Oklahoma City, OK, USA
[6]Cardiac Electrophysiology Department, University of California, San Francisco, CA, USA
[7]Cardiology Department, Veterans General Hospital, Taipei, Taiwan

Introduction

The initial hypotheses on AF pathogenesis date back to the early 1900s when the two main theories of focal activity and multiple reentry circuits were proposed. Despite extensive studies at both experimental and clinical level, significant open issues still remain and a unifying theory is lacking.

It is clear that the pathogenesis of AF is often multifaceted and the arrhythmia may develop in different pathologic conditions as well as in the normal heart. It is well recognized that increased atrial mass, decreased conduction velocity, and decreased atrial refractoriness with increased dispersion are all pro-fibrillatory factors. The onset and maintenance of AF, irrespective of the underlying mechanism, requires an event (trigger) that initiates the arrhythmia and the presence of a predisposing substrate that perpetuates it. Additional factors (e.g., inflammation or autonomic tone) may also cooperate as "modulators" in facilitating initiation or continuation of AF. Certain key points are summarized in the following.

Diseases associated with AF and the role of fibrosis

Although approximately 10% of AF patients have no evident cardiac disorder (so-called lone AF), the arrhythmia usually occurs in patients with SHD [1,2]. Hypertension, coronary heart disease, valvular heart disease,

Atrial Fibrillation Ablation, 2011 Update: The State of the Art based on the VeniceChart International Consensus Document, First Edition. Edited by Andrea Natale and Antonio Raviele.
© 2011 John Wiley & Sons, Ltd. Published 2011 by John Wiley & Sons, Ltd.

dilated cardiomyopathy, and heart failure are the most frequent pathological conditions associated with AF (Table 2.1) [3]. Other diseases causing AF include HCM, congenital heart disease, pericarditis, and left atrial myxoma. All the above diseases can cause atrial pressure and/or volume overload and lead to primary or secondary atrial interstitial fibrosis [3,4]. Noncardiac abnormalities, including metabolic disorders (diabetes, hyperthyroidism, and pheochromocytoma), pulmonary diseases (chronic obstructive pulmonary disease, obstructive sleep apnea, and postpulmonary surgery), excessive alcohol, and coffee drinking are all well known to predispose to AF. Atrial enlargement is often present in patients with AF, although it is difficult to establish if it represents the cause or the consequence of the arrhythmia. Atrial fibrosis and loss of myocardial tissue are common findings in patients with AF and the amount of fibrosis in the atria correlates with the persistence of AF [4], suggesting that atrial fibrosis results in structural remodeling to promote AF. Thus, fibrosis has an apparent clear impact in facilitating AF by reducing the conduction velocity and possibly creating areas of conduction block. As such, fibrosis may be either a substrate for AF (due to coexisting heart disease) or a result of fibrillating atria and part of the so-called structural remodeling [5]. However, increased amounts of fibrosis occur not only when AF is associated with other cardiac diseases [4,6] but also in patients with lone AF [6,7]. The mechanistic importance of fibrosis in the occurrence of AF is strongly supported by studies in animal models in which selective atrial fibrosis caused by overexpression of TGF-β1 increases AF vulnerability [8,9]. In addition, it has been demonstrated that activation of the renin–angiotensin system with increases in angiotensin II levels promotes formation of collagen [10–12]. Therefore, pharmacological inhibition of this system could represent a novel approach to counteract development of fibrosis and recurrence of AF [11,13,14]. This may explain the apparent benefit in the prevention of AF observed in many post hoc analyses of randomized controlled trials in which angiotensin-converting enzyme inhibitors or angiotensin receptor blockers have been compared with placebo [1].

Genetic factors and ion channel diseases

A number of studies provide irrefutable evidence for a genetic component in the case of lone AF, which develops in the absence of the traditional risk factors [15,16]. These studies showed a large heritable contribution in lone AF, suggesting a traditional monogenic syndrome with reduced penetrance. Several Mendelian loci for lone AF have been identified, although the specific gene has not as yet been identified in all cases [17,18].

Genetic linkage analyses have identified AF loci on chromosomes 10q22-24, [17] 6q14-16 [18], 5p13 [19], and 11p15.5 [20]. In the case of 11p15.5, the genetic defect involved heterozygous missense mutations in *KCNQ1*, resulting in gain of function of the *KCNQ1-KCNE1* and *KCNQ1-KCNE2* ion channels conducting the slowly activating delayed rectifier current, I_{Ks} [20].

Table 2.1 Causes of AF.

	Group	Factor/disease	Proposed mechanism
Substrate	Associated diseases causing atrial enlargement and fibrosis	Hypertension Valvular disease Coronary artery disease/ heart failure	• Increased profibrotic factors (TGFβ-1) • Increased atrial stretch
	Genetic—Mendelian disorders	Short QT syndrome	• KCNQ1:↑ I_{Ks} > ↓ERP • KCNH2: ↑ I_{Kr} >↓ ERP • KCNJ2: ↑ I_{K1} >↓ ERP • CACNA1C: ↓I_{ca}> ↓ ERP • CACNB2b: ↓I_{ca}> ↓ ERP • CACNA2D1: ↓I_{ca}> ↓ ERP
		Brugada syndrome	• SCN5A: ↓ I_{Na} • GPD1-L: ↓ I_{Na} • CACNA1C: ↓I_{Ca} • CACNB2b: ↓I_{ca} • SCN1B: ↓ I_{Na} • KCNE3: ↑ I_{to} • SCN3B: ↓ I_{Na} • CACNA2D1: ↓I_{Ca} • KCNJ8: ↑ I_{K-ATP}
		Long QT syndrome	• SCN5A: ↑ Late I_{Na} • ANKB:
		Nuclear pore component	NUP155: ↓ nuclear membrane permeability
		Other	• KCNA5 ↓ I_{Kur} • KCNE2: ↑ I_K • NPAA: ↑ NPA • KCNE5: ↑ I_{Ks} • ABCC9: ↑ I_{K-ATP}
	Genetic—somatic genetic defects	Connexin genes (mutations and promoter polymorphisms)	• GJA5: impaired electrical conduction
	Genetic mitochondrial DNA[a]	mtDNA4977 (nt8224-13501 deletion)	• Impaired energy substrate production leading to cell death and fibrosis

[a]Age-related accumulation of mutations and possible matrilineal transmission.

Gain-of-function mutations in *KCNE2* [21] and *KCNJ2* [22], encoding the inward rectifier potassium current (I_{K1}), have been associated with familial AF in two Chinese kindreds. Similar studies have associated human AF with genes coding (1) the α subunit of the $K_v1.5$ channel responsible for I_{Kur} (*KCNA5*), (2) the gap junctional protein Connexin40 (*GJA5*), (3) SUR2A, the ATP regulatory subunit of the cardiac K_{ATP} channel (*ABCC9*), and (4) *KCNE5* which co-associates with *KCNQ1* to form the I_{Ks} channel [23–27] (Table 2.1). Relatively rare forms of familial AF have also been associated with inherited channelopathies such as Brugada, long QT syndrome, and short QT syndrome as well as with cardiomyopathies [21,28–32] (Table 2.1). These are caused by mutations in one or more subunits of potassium, sodium, and calcium ion channel genes, as well as in a nuclear pore [33], anchoring protein [34], and natriuretic peptide gene [35].

Recent GWAS have identified a locus on chromosome 4q25. Although far from any obvious gene, the 4q45 locus is downstream from a paired-like homeodomain transcription factor 2 (*PITX2*) [36,37]. *Pitx2c* is expressed in the immediate postnatal period in the LA and PVs and binds to *Shox2*, suggesting that it directly represses the sinoatrial node genetic program [38,39]. This information has provided support for the role of *Pitx2c* as an atrial arrhythmia susceptibility gene. GWAS have also identified other loci including one within the *ZFHX3* gene on chromosome 16q22 and the *KCNN3* gene on 1q21 [40]. *KCNN3*, which encodes the small conductance calcium-activated potassium channel subfamily N, member 3 (SK3; $K_{Ca}2.3$), has also recently been associated with preterm (<37 weeks gestation) infant birth [41].

Genetic animal models have added to our understanding of the role of genetics in AF [42,43]. A *KCNE1* knockout mouse exhibits paroxysmal AF via a mechanism largely due to abbreviated ventricular repolarization [43]. Atria isolated from transgenic mice in which *KCNJ2* (Kir2.1) was overexpressed develops AF more readily and the rotors responsible for the maintenance of AF are faster and more stable as a result of the upregulation of I_{K1} [44,45]. A transgenic mouse overexpressing canine junctin in the heart develops cardiac enlargement, atrial fibrosis, bradycardia, and AF [46]. In knockout mice lacking Cx40, AF is readily induced by standard pacing protocols [47]. Finally, a mouse model that lacks I_{K-ACh} exhibits a reduced susceptibility to AF, supporting the benefit of I_{K-ACh} blockers as therapy for AF [48].

Despite great strides in recent years, the genetic basis for the majority of patients with AF remains elusive. Elucidation of the genetic factors contributing to the development of AF will no doubt advance our understanding of the etiologies of the disease and assist in identification of discrete clinical subtypes, thus improving diagnosis and the approach to therapy [49]. Although genetic screening for AF is an important target for research, it is as yet not indicated as a clinical test for patients with AF.

Electrophysiological mechanisms

General concepts

Increased automaticity and single and multiple circuit reentry can cause AF (Table 2.2). These mechanisms are not mutually exclusive and are probably variable according to the underlying pathogenesis. It is likely that areas of focal firing and areas of reentry are present simultaneously in varying degrees in the majority of patients. The degree of each may affect the frequency and duration of episodes and may account for the wide range of electrogram patterns (i.e., rapid, highly fractionated electrograms or slower organized electrograms) recorded at different sites in the atria at any given time. The principal factors leading to focal firing and/or reentry may differ between patients. For example, there may be differences between patients in the degree to which the length of a pause, the degree of calcium loading, or the degree of autonomic sensitivity combine to produce focal firing in the PV myocardium. Regardless, the onset and maintenance of the arrhythmia require both a trigger and a substrate (Table 2.2).

Trigger and AF sources

Recent observations have focused attention on the PVs as a source of ectopic activity-determining AF [2,50]. It is now widely accepted that the PVs are an important source of ectopic beats, that they are capable of initiating frequent paroxysms of AF, and that they could be eliminated by treatment with RFA [50,51]. As such PV isolation has become the gold standard of management in the clinical EP laboratory and is the recommended treatment in drug-refractory AF, which very effectively terminates most cases of paroxysmal AF [52].

Other anatomical structures that may also provide ectopic beats causing AF are the SVC, the vein of Marshall, the musculature of CS, the posterior wall of the LA and the left atrial appendage [53, 54]. Yet for AF to become sustained the presence of an atrial substrate capable of maintaining reentrant circuits is necessary. The demonstration that the isolation of ectopic focal discharges in the PVs can cure a significant proportion of patients with paroxysmal AF demonstrates the crucial pathophysiological importance of the LA–PV junction and the posterior wall of LA [55]. Unfortunately, the cellular mechanism(s) of such discharges has not been established with any degree of certainty. The mechanism could be microreentrant, triggered, or abnormally automatic. Similarly, reentry in the form of electrical waves rotating at high speed and generating fibrillatory conduction from one to the other atrium have been demonstrated to occur, at least experimentally, in both acute and chronic AF [56–58]. Consistent with such vortices, clinical studies have provided clear evidence for a hierarchical distribution of DFs between the left and the RA, supporting the idea that localized sources of sustained reentrant activity underlies the mechanism of many cases of paroxysmal AF [59–64], and even some cases of persistent/permanent AF [59–64].

Table 2.2 Triggers, sources, and modulating factors of AF.

	Group	Factor/disease	Proposed mechanism
Triggers	PVs, PLA, abnormal excitability	Focal activity Reentry	• Triggered activity, increased automaticity, and reentry due to short action potential; complex 3D atrial structure
	Non-PV foci	Vein of Marshall, CS, PLA, SVC, LAA	
AF sources	Rotors Focal	Left versus right atrial differences in ion channel distribution	• Left-to-right DF gradients Fibrillatory conduction
Modulating factors	Inflammation	Increased C-reactive protein	• Progressive APD shortening and dispersion of refractory periods
	Electrical remodeling	Reduced CaV1.2 (L-type calcium channel) expression	• Impaired excitability favoring both initiation and maintenance of AF
		Reduced NCX (sodium calcium exchanger) expression	
		Reduced Kv4.3 (transient outward current) expression	
		Increased K$^+$ channel beta subunit expression (minK and MiRp2) expression	
		Increased expression of TWIK-1, two-pores K$^+$ channel	
		Increased expression of Kir2.1	
	Structural Remodeling	Patchy atrial fibrosis, dilatation, increased compliance, heterogeneous impulse propagation and reduced contractility	• Myocyte dedifferentiation • Calcium dysregulation • Increased ECM protein deposition and turnover
	SNS/RAS	Increased parasympathetic tone and RAS pathway	• Reduced refractory period • Increased cell damage

A left-to-right difference in the density of the strong inward rectifier current, I_{K1}, may explain the DF gradient in patients with paroxysmal AF [65,66]. Nevertheless, as shown recently in an experimental model of autonomically mediated AF [67], the complexities of reentrant activity can be substantially exacerbated by their interaction with repetitive or intermittent focal activity, which strongly implicates dysfunctional calcium dynamics in the mechanism of some forms of AF [67,68]. As such, focal activity cannot be ruled out even in those cases in which the clear presence of rotors has been documented.

The third dimension

Clearly, the 3D anatomical structure of the atrial muscle is likely to be a crucial factor in determining the ultimate fibrillatory behavior (Table 2.2). It has been shown that the *crista terminalis* and the pectinate muscles are sites of preferential propagation whose frequency dependence enables disparity between endocardial and epicardial activation as well as reentry [69,70]. The 3D anatomy of the tissue is also responsible for the fragmentation of waves and conduction block. For instance, studies in isolated sheep hearts have shown that the interface between Bachmann's bundle and the branching pectinate muscles of the RAA show abrupt changes in their thickness and frequency-dependent sink-to-source mismatch [70]. Here, spatially distributed intermittent block of wavefronts makes the RA incapable of activating 1:1 in response to impulses traveling from the LA at frequencies higher than $\sim$6.8 Hz (so-called breakdown frequency), even if the input frequency is highly periodic [70]. High frequency stimulation of the PVs originates wavebreaks in areas of abrupt fiber orientation and wall thickness in the posterior wall of the LA [71].

Recently the substrate of long-standing persistent AF was analyzed in detail in 24 patients with SHD [72,73]. Extensive epicardial mapping of the right and left atria showed numerous narrow wavelets, separated by lines of conduction block, predominantly oriented parallel to the atrial muscle bundles. In a total of >4000 fibrillation maps, not a single reentrant circuit could be detected on the epicardium of the right and left atria (including the area between the PVs). In contrast, many fibrillation waves with a focal spread of activation were observed. These waves emerged at multiple sites, were distributed over the entire atrial wall, but as a rule were not repetitive and had no fixed coupling intervals. Previously, optical mapping of the right atrial epicardium of the isolated sheep heart during acute, sustained AF revealed that propagation was characterized by a combination of incomplete reentry, breakthrough patterns, and wave collisions [69]. Incomplete reentry occurred when waves propagated around thin lines of block and then terminated. Breakthrough patterns were frequent and their location and the lines of block during incomplete reentry were not randomly distributed but appeared to be related to preferential propagation in the underlying subendocardial muscle structures, suggesting repetitive transmural reentry. More recently, simultaneous endo-epicardial mapping in the goat provided strong confirmation of the existence of endo-epicardial dissociation during persistent AF [74]. It has been suggested that dissociation provides a constant source of new fibrillation waves for the epi-endocardial surfaces, which would offer an adequate explanation for the high persistence of AF in patients with SHD even in the absence of a focal or reentrant source [72]. If satisfactorily validated, such a 3D concept of the substrate of AF might explain why in the end-stage of structural atrial remodeling even the most extensive ablation procedure often fails to restore and maintain sinus rhythm.

Role of the autonomic tone
The role of parasympathetic and sympathetic tone as initiators of AF has been extensively studied in the past. Vagal stimulation shortens refractory period, and sympathetic stimulation increases calcium loading and automaticity. Combined, they cause pause-induced triggered activity in PV and atrial myocytes. The mechanism of triggered firing may relate to the combination of very short APD and increased calcium release during systole, leading to high intracellular calcium during and after repolarization. It has been proposed that the high calcium concentration activates the sodium/calcium exchanger (3 Na^+ ions move into the cell for each Ca^{++} ion extruded), leading to a net inward current, early afterdepolarizations and triggered firing [75–77]. Compared to atrial myocytes, PV myocytes have shorter APD and greater sensitivity to autonomic stimulation, which may explain the predominance of pause-induced focal firing in the PVs [78], and the interruption of focal firing by ablation of the autonomic GP. Interruption of nerves from the GP to the PVs may explain the frequent elimination of focal firing produced by PV isolation procedures during ablation therapy. These findings support the role of GP activity in the onset and perpetuation of AF, and may explain the success of early ablation studies targeting only the GP [79,80].

Structural and electrical remodeling
The process of AF self-perpetuation is called remodeling. Both structural and electrical remodeling can occur when AF profoundly impacts on the atrial tissue activating several pathways contributing to its maintenance [81–86] (Table 2.2). At the macroscopic level, AF causes atrial fibrosis, dilatation, increased compliance, and reduced contractility. Ultrastructural changes of myocytes (so-called dedifferentiation, because myocytes return to the fetal aspect) include increase in cell size, accumulation of glycogen, myolysis, alterations in connexin expression, changes in mitochondrial shape, and fragmentation of sarcoplasmic reticulum [5]. Interestingly, such changes are not uniform throughout the atria and therefore they may substantially contribute to electrical instability by creating further heterogeneity of the electrical properties. Electrical remodeling parallels the structural abnormalities and patchy fibrosis observed during AF. Progressive shortening and dispersion of refractory periods are the main changes occurring during AF [81].

Role of inflammation

Clinical studies have provided evidence for a role of inflammation as a contributing factor in the pathophysiology of AF, particularly in patients with persistent AF [87,88]. In fact, multiple associations have been reported between AF vulnerability and increased circulating levels of cytokines, C-reactive protein, complement [88–90] and, importantly, the activation state of leukocytes [7,91,92]. However, it remains unclear whether an inflammatory phenotype is mechanistically related, either directly or indirectly, to the initiation and progression of AF. One reasonable possibility is that inflammation contributes to AF through the remodeling of the ECM and the generation of atrial fibrosis. Data in the literature suggest that increased deposition and turnover of ECM proteins leading to atrial fibrosis is accelerated after exposure to inflammatory cytokines, C-reactive protein, and complement [93]. These effects seem to be mediated through activation of MMPs, which are enzymes that are important in ECM turnover and have been strongly linked to ECM remodeling in AF [94]. A recent study investigated the role of the leukocyte-derived heme MPO, which is an essential regulator of MMP activity [95], in the initiation and perpetuation of AF and its contribution to atrial fibrosis [96]. The results demonstrated that atrial accumulation of MPO was accompanied by augmented fibrosis in mice and humans with AF and strongly suggested that MPO is intimately involved in the pathophysiology of AF [96]. The data of that study provided important evidence on the role of inflammation in fibrosis associated with AF and proposed that MPO may serve as a potential new target of AF treatment [97]. It has been shown that tumor necrosis factor-α alters calcium handling and increases arrhythmogenesis in PV cardiomyocytes [98]. On the other hand heat stress seems to prevent AF [99] and increases calcium currents as well as the expression of SERCA2a, sodium calcium exchanger and heat shock proteins as well as electrophysiological properties in atrial myocytes [100]. Finally, it was reported recently that CD36 levels in monocytes were independently correlated with AF and could predict the outcome after the catheter ablation [101]. Altogether these data AF support the role of intracellular calcium dysregulation, inflammation, and fibrosis as contributing factors in AF.

References

1. Fuster V, Ryden LE, Cannom DS, et al. ACC/AHA/ESC 2006 Guidelines for the Management of Patients with Atrial Fibrillation: A report of the American College of Cardiology/American Heart Association Task Force on Practice Guidelines and the European Society of Cardiology Committee for Practice Guidelines (Writing Committee to Revise the 2001 Guidelines for the Management of Patients With Atrial Fibrillation): Developed in collaboration with the European Heart Rhythm Association and the Heart Rhythm Society. Circulation 2006; 114:e257–354.
2. Calkins H, Brugada J, Packer DL, et al. HRS/EHRA/ECAS expert Consensus Statement on catheter and surgical ablation of atrial fibrillation: Recommendations for

personnel, policy, procedures and follow-up. A report of the Heart Rhythm Society (HRS) Task Force on catheter and surgical ablation of atrial fibrillation. Heart Rhythm 2007; 4:816–861.

3. Benjamin EJ, Chen PS, Bild DE, et al. Prevention of atrial fibrillation: Report from a national heart, lung, and blood institute workshop. Circulation 2009; 119: 606–618.

4. Xu J, Cui G, Esmailian F, et al. Atrial extracellular matrix remodeling and the maintenance of atrial fibrillation. Circulation 2004; 109:363–368.

5. Ausma J, Wijffels M, Thone F, Wouters L, Allessie M, Borgers M. Structural changes of atrial myocardium due to sustained atrial fibrillation in the goat. Circulation 1997; 96:3157–3163.

6. Boldt A, Wetzel U, Lauschke J, et al. Fibrosis in left atrial tissue of patients with atrial fibrillation with and without underlying mitral valve disease. Heart 2004; 90:400–405.

7. Frustaci A, Chimenti C, Bellocci F, Morgante E, Russo MA, Maseri A. Histological substrate of atrial biopsies in patients with lone atrial fibrillation. Circulation 1997; 96:1180–1184.

8. Nakajima H, Nakajima HO, Salcher O, et al. Atrial but not ventricular fibrosis in mice expressing a mutant transforming growth factor-beta(1) transgene in the heart. Circ Res 2000; 86:571–579.

9. Verheule S, Sato T, Everett Tt, et al. Increased vulnerability to atrial fibrillation in transgenic mice with selective atrial fibrosis caused by overexpression of TGF-beta1. Circ Res 2004; 94:1458–1465.

10. Tharaux PL, Chatziantoniou C, Fakhouri F, Dussaule JC. Angiotensin II activates collagen I gene through a mechanism involving the MAP/ER kinase pathway. Hypertension 2000; 36:330–336.

11. Chen YJ, Chen YC, Tai CT, Yeh HI, Lin CI, Chen SA. Angiotensin II and angiotensin II receptor blocker modulate the arrhythmogenic activity of pulmonary veins. Br J Pharmacol 2006; 147:12–22.

12. Lu YY, Chen YC, Kao YH, Wu TJ, Chen SA, Chen YJ. Extracellular matrix of collagen modulates intracellular calcium handling and electrophysiological characteristics of HL-1 cardiomyocytes with activation of angiotensin II type 1 receptor. J Card Fail 2011; 17:82–90.

13. Khan R, Sheppard R. Fibrosis in heart disease: Understanding the role of transforming growth factor-beta in cardiomyopathy, valvular disease and arrhythmia. Immunology 2006; 118:10–24.

14. Sakabe M, Fujiki A, Nishida K, et al. Enalapril preserves sinus node function in a canine atrial fibrillation model induced by rapid atrial pacing. J Cardiovasc Electrophysiol 2005; 16:1209–1214.

15. Darbar D, Herron KJ, Ballew JD, et al. Familial atrial fibrillation is a genetically heterogeneous disorder. J Am Coll Cardiol 2003; 41:2185–2192.

16. Ellinor PT, Lunetta KL, Glazer NL, et al. Common variants in KCNN3 are associated with lone atrial fibrillation. Nat Genet 2010; 42:240–244.

17. Brugada R, Tapscott T, Czernuszewicz GZ, et al. Identification of a genetic locus for familial atrial fibrillation. N Engl J Med 1997; 336:905–911.

18. Ellinor PT, Shin JT, Moore RK, Yoerger DM, MacRae CA. Locus for atrial fibrillation maps to chromosome 6q14–16. Circulation 2003; 107:2880–2883.

19. Oberti C, Wang L, Li L, et al. Genome-wide linkage scan identifies a novel genetic locus on chromosome 5p13 for neonatal atrial fibrillation associated with sudden death and variable cardiomyopathy. Circulation 2004; 110:3753–3759.

20. Chen YH, Xu SJ, Bendahhou S, et al. KCNQ1 gain-of-function mutation in familial atrial fibrillation. Science 2003; 299:251–254.

21. Yang Y, Xia M, Jin Q, et al. Identification of a KCNE2 gain-of-function mutation in patients with familial atrial fibrillation. Am J Hum Genet 2004; 75:899–905.

22. Xia M, Jin Q, Bendahhou S, et al. A Kir2.1 gain-of-function mutation underlies familial atrial fibrillation. Biochem Biophys Res Commun 2005; 332:1012–1019.

23. Olson TM, Alekseev AE, Liu XK, et al. Kv1.5 channelopathy due to KCNA5 loss-of-function mutation causes human atrial fibrillation. Hum Mol Genet 2006; 15: 2185–2191.

24. Gollob MH, Jones DL, Krahn AD, et al. Somatic mutations in the connexin 40 gene (GJA5) in atrial fibrillation. N Engl J Med 2006; 354:2677–2688.

25. Olson TM, Alekseev AE, Moreau C, et al. KATP channel mutation confers risk for vein of Marshall adrenergic atrial fibrillation. Nat Clin Pract Cardiovasc Med 2007; 4:110–116.

26. Ravn LS, Aizawa Y, Pollevick GD, et al. Gain of function in IKs secondary to a mutation in KCNE5 associated with atrial fibrillation. Heart Rhythm 2008; 5:427–435.

27. Antzelevitch C, Barajas-Martinez H. A gain-of-function I(K-ATP) mutation and its role in sudden cardiac death associated with J-wave syndromes. Heart Rhythm 2010; 7:1472–1474.

28. Schulze-Bahr E, Eckardt L, Breithardt G, et al. Sodium channel gene (SCN5A) mutations in 44 index patients with Brugada syndrome: Different incidences in familial and sporadic disease. Hum Mutat 2003; 21:651–652.

29. Antzelevitch C, Pollevick GD, Cordeiro JM, et al. Loss-of-function mutations in the cardiac calcium channel underlie a new clinical entity characterized by ST-segment elevation, short QT intervals, and sudden cardiac death. Circulation 2007; 115:442–449.

30. Watanabe H, Koopmann TT, Le Scouarnec S, et al. Sodium channel beta1 subunit mutations associated with Brugada syndrome and cardiac conduction disease in humans. J Clin Invest 2008; 118:2260–2268.

31. Brugada R, Hong K, Dumaine R, et al. Sudden death associated with short-QT syndrome linked to mutations in HERG. Circulation 2004; 109:30–35.

32. Priori SG, Pandit SV, Rivolta I, et al. A novel form of short QT syndrome (SQT3) is caused by a mutation in the KCNJ2 gene. Circ Res 2005; 96:800–807.

33. Zhang X, Chen S, Yoo S, et al. Mutation in nuclear pore component NUP155 leads to atrial fibrillation and early sudden cardiac death. Cell 2008; 135:1017–1027.

34. Abriel H. Cardiac sodium channel Na(v)1.5 and interacting proteins: Physiology and pathophysiology. J Mol Cell Cardiol 2010; 48:2–11.

35. Roberts JD, Davies RW, Lubitz SA, et al. Evaluation of non-synonymous NPPA single nucleotide polymorphisms in atrial fibrillation. Europace 2010; 12:1078–1083.

36. Kaab S, Darbar D, van Noord C, et al. Large scale replication and meta-analysis of variants on chromosome 4q25 associated with atrial fibrillation. Eur Heart J 2009; 30:813–819.

37. Gudbjartsson DF, Arnar DO, Helgadottir A, et al. Variants conferring risk of atrial fibrillation on chromosome 4q25. Nature 2007; 448:353–357.

38. Franco D, Campione M. The role of Pitx2 during cardiac development. Linking left-right signaling and congenital heart diseases. Trends Cardiovasc Med 2003; 13: 157–163.

39. Wang J, Klysik E, Sood S, Johnson RL, Wehrens XH, Martin JF. Pitx2 prevents susceptibility to atrial arrhythmias by inhibiting left-sided pacemaker specification. Proc Natl Acad Sci USA 2010; 107:9753–9758.

40. Benjamin EJ, Rice KM, Arking DE, et al. Variants in ZFHX3 are associated with atrial fibrillation in individuals of European ancestry. Nat Genet 2009; 41:879–881.
41. Day LJ, Schaa KL, Ryckman KK, et al. Single-Nucleotide Polymorphisms in the KCNN3 Gene Associate With Preterm Birth. Reprod Sci 2011.
42. Olgin JE, Verheule S. Transgenic and knockout mouse models of atrial arrhythmias. Cardiovasc Res 2002; 54:280–286.
43. Temple J, Frias P, Rottman J, et al. Atrial fibrillation in KCNE1-null mice. Circ Res 2005; 97:62–69.
44. Li J, McLerie M, Lopatin AN. Transgenic upregulation of IK1 in the mouse heart leads to multiple abnormalities of cardiac excitability. Am J Physiol Heart Circ Physiol 2004; 287:H2790–2802.
45. Noujaim SF, Pandit SV, Berenfeld O, et al. Up-regulation of the inward rectifier K+ current (I K1) in the mouse heart accelerates and stabilizes rotors. J Physiol 2007; 578:315–326.
46. Hong CS, Cho MC, Kwak YG, et al. Cardiac remodeling and atrial fibrillation in transgenic mice overexpressing junctin. FASEB J 2002; 16:1310–1312.
47. Hagendorff A, Schumacher B, Kirchhoff S, Luderitz B, Willecke K. Conduction disturbances and increased atrial vulnerability in Connexin40-deficient mice analyzed by transesophageal stimulation. Circulation 1999; 99:1508–1515.
48. Milan DJ, MacRae CA. Animal models for arrhythmias. Cardiovasc Res 2005; 67:426–437.
49. Sabeh MK, Macrae CA. The genetics of atrial fibrillation. Curr Opin Cardiol 2010; 25: 186- 191.
50. Haissaguerre M, Jais P, Shah DC, et al. Spontaneous initiation of atrial fibrillation by ectopic beats originating in the pulmonary veins. N Engl J Med 1998; 339: 659–666.
51. Oral H. What have we learned about atrial arrhythmias from ablation of chronic atrial fibrillation? Heart Rhythm 2008; 5:S36–39.
52. Dewire J, Calkins H. State-of-the-art and emerging technologies for atrial fibrillation ablation. Nat Rev Cardiol 2010; 7:129–138.
53. Lin WS, Tai CT, Hsieh MH, et al. Catheter ablation of paroxysmal atrial fibrillation initiated by non-pulmonary vein ectopy. Circulation 2003; 107:3176–3183.
54. Di Biase L, Burkhardt JD, Mohanty P, et al. Left atrial appendage: an underrecognized trigger site of atrial fibrillation. Circulation 2010; 122:109–18.
55. Oral H, Chugh A, Good E, et al. Randomized comparison of encircling and nonencircling left atrial ablation for chronic atrial fibrillation. Heart Rhythm 2005; 2: 1165–1172.
56. Mandapati R, Skanes A, Chen J, Berenfeld O, Jalife J. Stable microreentrant sources as a mechanism of atrial fibrillation in the isolated sheep heart. Circulation 2000; 101:194–199.
57. Mansour M, Mandapati R, Berenfeld O, Chen J, Samie FH, Jalife J. Left-to-right gradient of atrial frequencies during acute atrial fibrillation in the isolated sheep heart. Circulation 2001; 103:2631–2636.
58. Jalife J. Experimental and clinical AF mechanisms: Bridging the divide. J Interv Card Electrophysiol 2003; 9:85–92.
59. Lazar S, Dixit S, Marchlinski FE, Callans DJ, Gerstenfeld EP. Presence of left-to-right atrial frequency gradient in paroxysmal but not persistent atrial fibrillation in humans. Circulation 2004; 110:3181–3186.

60. Sahadevan J, Ryu K, Peltz L, et al. Epicardial mapping of chronic atrial fibrillation in patients: Preliminary observations. Circulation 2004; 110:3293–3299.

61. Sanders P, Berenfeld O, Hocini M, et al. Spectral analysis identifies sites of high-frequency activity maintaining atrial fibrillation in humans. Circulation 2005; 112: 789–797.

62. Dibs SR, Ng J, Arora R, Passman RS, Kadish AH, Goldberger JJ. Spatiotemporal characterization of atrial activation in persistent human atrial fibrillation: Multisite electrogram analysis and surface electrocardiographic correlations–a pilot study. Heart Rhythm 2008; 5:686–693.

63. Atienza F, Almendral J, Moreno J, et al. Activation of inward rectifier potassium channels accelerates atrial fibrillation in humans: Evidence for a reentrant mechanism. Circulation 2006; 114:2434–2442.

64. Atienza F, Almendral J, Jalife J, et al. Real-time dominant frequency mapping and ablation of dominant frequency sites in atrial fibrillation with left-to-right frequency gradients predicts long-term maintenance of sinus rhythm. Heart Rhythm 2009; 6:33–40.

65. Jalife J, Berenfeld O, Mansour M. Mother rotors and fibrillatory conduction: A mechanism of atrial fibrillation. Cardiovasc Res 2002; 54:204–216.

66. Voigt N, Trausch A, Knaut M, et al. Left-to-Right Atrial Inward-Rectifier Potassium Current Gradients in Patients with Paroxysmal Versus Chronic Atrial Fibrillation. Circ Arrhythm Electrophysiol 2010; 1:472–480.

67. Yamazaki M, Vaquero LM, Hou L, et al. Mechanisms of stretch-induced atrial fibrillation in the presence and the absence of adrenocholinergic stimulation: Interplay between rotors and focal discharges. Heart Rhythm 2009; 6:1009–1017.

68. Chou CC, Nguyen BL, Tan AY, et al. Intracellular calcium dynamics and acetylcholine-induced triggered activity in the pulmonary veins of dogs with pacing-induced heart failure. Heart Rhythm 2008; 5:1170–1177.

69. Gray RA, Pertsov AM, Jalife J. Incomplete reentry and epicardial breakthrough patterns during atrial fibrillation in the sheep heart. Circulation 1996; 94:2649–2661.

70. Berenfeld O, Zaitsev AV, Mironov SF, Pertsov AM, Jalife J. Frequency-dependent breakdown of wave propagation into fibrillatory conduction across the pectinate muscle network in the isolated sheep right atrium. Circ Res 2002; 90:1173–1180.

71. Klos M, Calvo D, Yamazaki M, et al. Atrial septopulmonary bundle of the posterior left atrium provides a substrate for atrial fibrillation initiation in a model of vagally mediated pulmonary vein tachycardia of the structurally normal heart. Circ Arrhythm Electrophysiol 2008; 1:175–183.

72. Allessie MA, de Groot NM, Houben RP, et al. Electropathological substrate of long-standing persistent atrial fibrillation in patients with structural heart disease: Longitudinal dissociation. Circ Arrhythm Electrophysiol 2010; 3:606–615.

73. de Groot NM, Houben RP, Smeets JL, et al. Electropathological substrate of longstanding persistent atrial fibrillation in patients with structural heart disease: Epicardial breakthrough. Circulation 2010; 122:1674–1682.

74. Eckstein J, Maesen B, Linz D, et al. Time course and mechanisms of endo-epicardial electrical dissociation during atrial fibrillation in the goat. Cardiovasc Res 2010; 1:816–824.

75. Patterson E, Po SS, Scherlag BJ, Lazzara R. Triggered firing in pulmonary veins initiated by in vitro autonomic nerve stimulation. Heart Rhythm 2005; 2:624–631.

76. Patterson E, Lazzara R, Szabo B, et al. Sodium-calcium exchange initiated by the Ca2+ transient: An arrhythmia trigger within pulmonary veins. J Am Coll Cardiol 2006; 47:1196–1206.

77. Burashnikov A, Antzelevitch C. Reinduction of atrial fibrillation immediately after termination of the arrhythmia is mediated by late phase 3 early afterdepolarization-induced triggered activity. Circulation 2003; 107:2355–2360.

78. Patterson E, Jackman WM, Beckman KJ, et al. Spontaneous pulmonary vein firing in man: Relationship to tachycardia-pause early afterdepolarizations and triggered arrhythmia in canine pulmonary veins in vitro. J Cardiovasc Electrophysiol 2007; 18:1067–1075.

79. Lemery R, Birnie D, Tang AS, Green M, Gollob M. Feasibility study of endocardial mapping of ganglionated plexuses during catheter ablation of atrial fibrillation. Heart Rhythm 2006; 3:387–396.

80. Pokushalov E, Romanov A, Artyomenko S, Turov A, Shirokova N, Katritsis DG. Left atrial ablation at the anatomic areas of ganglionated plexi for paroxysmal atrial fibrillation. Pacing Clin Electrophysiol 2010; 33:1231–1238.

81. Wijffels MC, Kirchhof CJ, Dorland R, Allessie MA. Atrial fibrillation begets atrial fibrillation. A study in awake chronically instrumented goats. Circulation 1995; 92:1954–1968.

82. Morillo CA, Klein GJ, Jones DL, Guiraudon CM. Chronic rapid atrial pacing. Structural, functional, and electrophysiological characteristics of a new model of sustained atrial fibrillation. Circulation 1995; 91:1588–1595.

83. Ohki R, Yamamoto K, Ueno S, et al. Gene expression profiling of human atrial myocardium with atrial fibrillation by DNA microarray analysis. Int J Cardiol 2005; 102:233–238.

84. Nattel S, Shiroshita-Takeshita A, Brundel BJ, Rivard L. Mechanisms of atrial fibrillation: Lessons from animal models. Prog Cardiovasc Dis 2005; 48:9–28.

85. Gaborit N, Steenman M, Lamirault G, et al. Human atrial ion channel and transporter subunit gene-expression remodeling associated with valvular heart disease and atrial fibrillation. Circulation 2005; 112:471–481.

86. El-Armouche A, Boknik P, Eschenhagen T, et al. Molecular determinants of altered Ca2+ handling in human chronic atrial fibrillation. Circulation 2006; 114:670–680.

87. Chung MK, Martin DO, Sprecher D, et al. C-reactive protein elevation in patients with atrial arrhythmias: Inflammatory mechanisms and persistence of atrial fibrillation. Circulation 2001; 104:2886–2891.

88. Aviles RJ, Martin DO, Apperson-Hansen C, Houghtaling PL, et al. Inflammation as a risk factor for atrial fibrillation. Circulation 2003; 108:3006–3010.

89. Sata N, Hamada N, Horinouchi T, et al. C-reactive protein and atrial fibrillation. Is inflammation a consequence or a cause of atrial fibrillation? Jpn Heart J 2004; 45:441–445.

90. Conway DS, Buggins P, Hughes E, Lip GY. Prognostic significance of raised plasma levels of interleukin-6 and C-reactive protein in atrial fibrillation. Am Heart J 2004; 148:462–466.

91. Fontes ML, Mathew JP, Rinder HM, Zelterman D, Smith BR, Rinder CS. Atrial fibrillation after cardiac surgery/cardiopulmonary bypass is associated with monocyte activation. Anesth Analg 2005; 101:17–23.

92. Nakamura Y, Nakamura K, Fukushima-Kusano K, et al. Tissue factor expression in atrial endothelia associated with nonvalvular atrial fibrillation: Possible involvement in intracardiac thrombogenesis. Thromb Res 2003; 111:137–142.

93. Issac TT, Dokainish H, Lakkis NM. Role of inflammation in initiation and perpetuation of atrial fibrillation: A systematic review of the published data. J Am Coll Cardiol 2007; 50:2021–2028.

94. Chen CL, Huang SK, Lin JL, et al. Upregulation of matrix metalloproteinase-9 and tissue inhibitors of metalloproteinases in rapid atrial pacing-induced atrial fibrillation. J Mol Cell Cardiol 2008; 45:742–753.

95. Fu X, Kassim SY, Parks WC, Heinecke JW. Hypochlorous acid generated by myeloperoxidase modifies adjacent tryptophan and glycine residues in the catalytic domain of matrix metalloproteinase-7 (matrilysin): An oxidative mechanism for restraining proteolytic activity during inflammation. J Biol Chem 2003; 278:28403–28409.

96. Rudolph V, Andrie RP, Rudolph TK, et al. Myeloperoxidase acts as a profibrotic mediator of atrial fibrillation. Nat Med 2010; 16:470–474.

97. Rudolph V, Baldus S. Myeloperoxidase for guiding therapy for acute cardiac decompensation? It's heart to tell. Clin Chem 2010; 56:881–882.

98. Lee SH, Chen YC, Chen YJ, et al. Tumor necrosis factor-alpha alters calcium handling and increases arrhythmogenesis of pulmonary vein cardiomyocytes. Life Sci 2007; 80:1806–1815.

99. Brundel BJ, Shiroshita-Takeshita A, Qi X, et al. Induction of heat shock response protects the heart against atrial fibrillation. Circ Res 2006; 99:1394–1402.

100. Chen YC, Kao YH, Huang CF, Cheng CC, Chen YJ, Chen SA. Heat stress responses modulate calcium regulations and electrophysiological characteristics in atrial myocytes. J Mol Cell Cardiol 2010; 48:781–788.

101. Hu YF, Yeh HI, Tsao HM, et al. The Impact of the Circulating Monocyte CD36 Level on Atrial Fibrillation and the Subsequent Catheter Ablation. Heart Rhythm 2010; 8:650–656.

CHAPTER 3

Techniques and technologies for atrial fibrillation catheter ablation

Karl H. Kuck[1], Pedro Adragao[2], David J. Burkhardt[3], Pierre Jaïs[4], David Keane[5], Hiroshi Nakagawa[6], Robert A. Schweikert[7], Jasbir Sra[8], Vivek Y. Reddy[9]

[1]Cardiology Department, Asklepios Klinik St. Georg, Hamburg, Germany
[2]Cardiology Department, Hospital Santa Cruz, Carnaxide, Portugal
[3]Texas Cardiac Arrhythmia Institute, St. David's Medical Center, Austin, TX, USA
[4]Cardiology Department, Hôpital Haut-Lévêque, CHU de Bordeaux, Bordeaux, France
[5]Cardiology Department, St. Vincent's University Hospital, Dublin, Ireland
[6]Heart Rhythm Institute, University of Oklahoma Health Sciences Center, Oklahoma City, OK, USA
[7]Cardiology Department, Akron General Medical Center, Akron, OH, USA
[8]Aurora Cardiovascular Services, Aurora Sinai Medical Center, Milwaukee, WI, USA
[9]Cardiac Arrhythmia Department, The Zena and Michael A. Wiener Cardiovascular Institute, New York, NY, USA

The optimal method and tools for catheter ablation of AF have been much debated. At present, multiple approaches have been developed for catheter ablation of AF reporting similar success rates particularly in patients with paroxysmal and persistent AF. The current techniques focus on the elimination of mechanisms involved in the initiation and maintenance of AF, which are essentially represented by triggers—PVs and non-PV foci—and substrate (autonomic and electrophysiologic), as schematically shown in Figures 3.1 and 3.2. It should be recognized that although the techniques and endpoints of AF catheter ablation may differ significantly among centers, the resulting lesion set may be similar. This reflects the concept that complete isolation of the PVs and application of the lesion set proximal to the junction of the LA and tube-like portion of the PV are considered necessary by most techniques. The different approaches proposed for catheter ablation of AF include PVI, electrogram-based ablation or CFAE ablation, linear lesions, autonomic GP ablation, and sequential ablation strategy. The PVI comprises segmental/ostial PV ablation, circumferential PV ablation, and circumferential/ antral PVI. As these various techniques have evolved, new tools and technologies have been developed in an attempt to improve the efficacy and safety of catheter ablation of AF.

Atrial Fibrillation Ablation, 2011 Update: The State of the Art based on the VeniceChart International Consensus Document, First Edition. Edited by Andrea Natale and Antonio Raviele.
© 2011 John Wiley & Sons, Ltd. Published 2011 by John Wiley & Sons, Ltd.

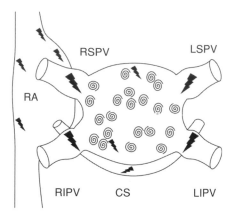

Figure 3.1 The current technologies focus on the elimination of mechanisms involved in the initiation and maintenance of AF, which are represented by triggers from and outside the pulmonary veins and substrate modification. The schematic shows triggering foci at the four pulmonary veins (RSPV, LSPV, RIPV, LIPV), CS, septum, and RA.

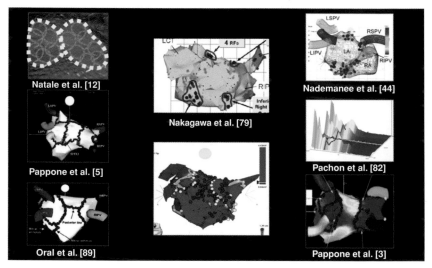

Figure 3.2 Evolving techniques for catheter ablation of AF (see the text for details).

PV isolation

"PVI" is a term that has been used to describe the electrical isolation of the PV from the adjacent LA. This has been almost universally accepted as the best endpoint for AF catheter ablation. The techniques and tools for AF catheter ablation have evolved substantially over the years since the early approach targeting the "focal triggers" within the PVs (Figure 3.3, Table 3.1). This early technique was associated with poor efficacy and a substantial risk of serious complications, notably PV stenosis. This was the major impetus for AF catheter ablation to evolve into an empirical approach with PVI. The various techniques outlined below reflect the ongoing progression of the tools and techniques for PVI as further experience and data were acquired over time.

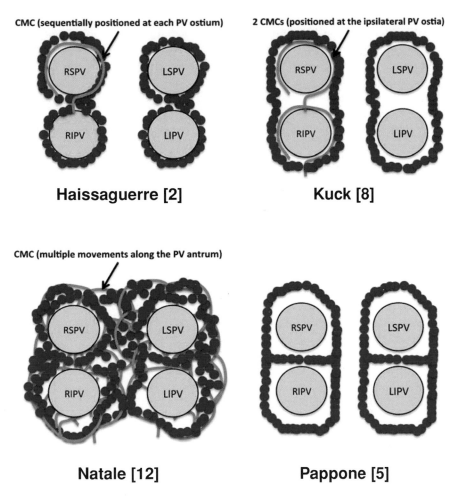

Figure 3.3 Different techniques of PVI.

Table 3.1 Different techniques for PV ablation.

Authors	Year	Ostium	Antrum	Imaging	Isolation verified
Haïssaguerre [2]	2000	Yes	No	PV angiography	Yes
Natale [12]	2003	No	Yes	ICE	Yes
Pappone [5]	2004	_[a]	_[a]	3D EAM + CT	No
Kuck [8]	2004	Yes	No	PV angiography	Yes[a]

Note: A CMC (two catheters in the technique by Kuck) is used for verification of PVI.
[a]Wide circumferential lines around the PVs.

The overriding course of development of the PVI technique has been a move from a distal location of ablation within the PVs to a much more proximal location within the LA near the PVs.

In whatever manner PVI is performed, electrical isolation of the PVs can be assessed in a variety of methods with various tools. However, the most commonly employed method is with the use of a CMC. This catheter can be deployed to the antrum, ostium or within the PV itself to assess the extent and location of electrical isolation. Such isolation can be determined by "entrance block" into the PV during sinus rhythm or atrial arrhythmia, and also by "exit block" with the use of stimulation (pacing) techniques within the PV. Other multielectrode systems have been developed to attempt to improve upon the CMC, such as multielectrode arrays. Other methods to assess for electrical isolation of the PV include the use of voltage mapping, as with 3D electroanatomical mapping systems.

Segmental/ostial PV isolation

A truly segmental PVI requires ablation inside the vein or very close to the output into the atrium [1,2]. It is now appreciated that ablation in the PVs themselves needs to be avoided as much as possible, primarily due to concern for development of PV stenosis. Consequently, the current emphasis is to ablate more atrially, which requires more extensive atrial ablation, often circumferentially as outlined in the techniques to follow. Therefore, the segmental/ostial PVI technique in the strictest sense has generally fallen out of favor, but remains of historical interest in the progression of the PVI technique. For segmental ostial PVI, a CMC of variable diameter (15–25 mm) is inserted into the LA through a long introducer via the transseptal route and is positioned sequentially at the ostia of the four PVs [2]. The ablation catheter is positioned at the ostium of the vein on the atrial side; a series of segmental lesions are then created until isolation of the vein can be demonstrated by disappearance of the venous potentials on the CMC (i.e., entrance block). Ablation can be performed in sinus rhythm or during AF. The literature data display complete agreement as to the need to achieve isolation of all four PVs.

Circumferential PV ablation

Circumferential PV ablation using 3D electroanatomical mapping was initially described by Pappone et al. [3,4]. Initially, the lesion set was limited to wide (>0.5 cm outside PV ostia) circumferential lesions around and outside the PV ostia but over time it was modified with wider (1–2 cm outside PV ostia) circumferential lesions, additional posterior lines connecting the PVs, the mitral isthmus line, and abolition of the evoked vagal reflexes, in order to increase the amount of substrate included in the ablation schema and in order to prevent recurrences of atrial tachycardia (Figure 3.4) [5,6]. RF energy is applied continuously on the planned circumferential lines, as the catheter is gradually dragged along the line, often in a to-and-fro fashion over a point.

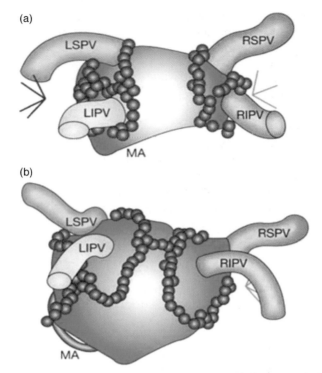

Figure 3.4 Evolution of circumferential PVI over time. Initially the lesion set was limited around and outside the PV ostia (a) but was later modified with wider circumferential lesions and additional lines connecting the PVs and the mitral isthmus to the inferior PV (b).

Successful lesion creation at each point is considered to have taken place when the local bipolar voltage has decreased by 90% or to less than 0.05 mV. The same ablation schema can be used when ablating paroxysmal, persistent, and long-lasting persistent AF.

A low complication rate has been reported with this technique.

This technique as initially designed did not involve verification of PVI, although electroanatomical 3D mapping techniques were subsequently employed to document voltage data to infer PVI. Many other centers have adopted this technique, some of which have added circular mapping to verify PV electrical isolation.

Circumferential/antral PVI

The key to this technique for PVI is delivery of the ablation lesions to the vestibule or "antrum" of the PV, which is the funnel-shaped portion of the LA (or perhaps more accurately the PV) that is proximal to the PV–LA junction or so-called ostium. The antrum includes the entire posterior wall and extends anteriorly to the right PVs on the septum (Figure 3.5). Defining this region during the ablation procedure can be monitored by various tools,

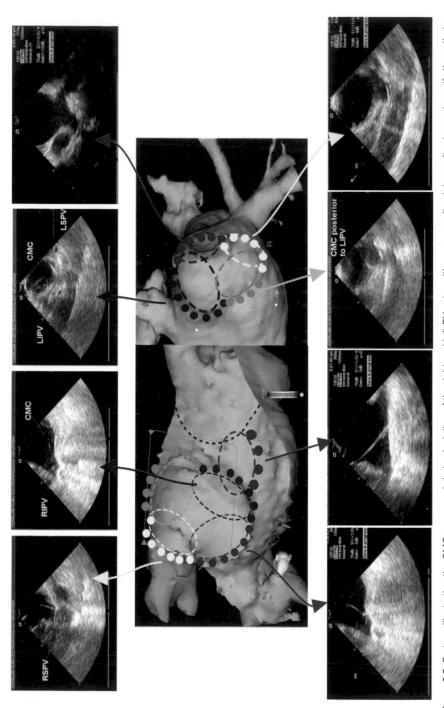

Figure 3.5 Cartoon illustrating the CMC movement during isolation of the right and left PV antra with corresponding intracardiac image to verify the catheter position. Dashed circles represent the CMC and dots represent the RFA delivered at the respective CMC position.

according to operator preference. Selective pulmonary venography is used by many centers to define the relevant anatomy. ICE has been increasingly used by many centers due to its ease of use and better capability to define the left atrial and proximal PV anatomy. ICE can also localize catheter position, and this is considered by some operators as crucial for this technique for correct positioning of the CMC at the antrum of the PVs. Such ICE guidance during PVI has been shown to reduce PV stenosis, for example [7]. However, cost is a limiting factor for the use of this technology at many centers. Computerized 3D mapping and navigation techniques (Carto, NavX, etc.) may be used to help define the relevant anatomy and provide a means of nonfluoroscopic catheter guidance. These techniques might be made more anatomically accurate by registration with other imaging techniques such as MR or CT, but the registration process remains tedious and fraught with the potential for inaccuracies if not performed with extreme precision. Technologies to perform "near real time" imaging in the EP laboratory, such as with rotational angiography, are available and might help to address some of the shortcomings of preprocedural imaging, but to date are still not sufficiently effective to result in widespread adoption.

The use of a multipolar CMC for PVI procedures has become incredibly widespread. One technique involves the use of two CMCs to achieve PVI [8]. The intracardiac echo-guided PV antrum isolation technique was developed primarily by the Natale group [9], and has been associated with outstanding efficacy and safety. The goal of this technique is to ensure that the ablation lesions are delivered outside the PVs at the region of the antrum. Typically, due to the very proximal region of delivery of ablation lesions, a circumferential lesion set is required.

For the CMC guided ablation technique, one or two CMCs are placed within the ipsilateral superior and inferior PVs or within the superior and inferior branches of a common PV during RF delivery. RF ablation is applied until the maximal local electrogram amplitude decreases by $\geq 90\%$. RF ablation is performed 1–2 cm outside the PV ostia, as defined by angiography, ICE, MR, or CT imaging. The endpoint is absence or dissociation of all PV potentials documented by CMC(s) within the ipsilateral superior and inferior PVs.

There have been reports of comparisons of various techniques for PVI as well as with other ablation strategies, either as an adjunct to PVI or as a standalone procedure [10,11]. From the available data, it appears that PVI remains quite important to the success of AF catheter ablation.

RF ablation catheter technologies might include standard tip (e.g., 4 mm), large tip (e.g., 8 mm), and closed or open irrigation. With the use of nonirrigated or closed-irrigation ablation catheter technologies, many centers employed ICE during lesion delivery to assess for the formation of microbubbles [12]. Although controversial to some, there is reasonable data and experience to indicate that such microbubbles represent tissue overheating [13]. As techniques moved away from the arguably less effective nonirrigated ablation catheter technologies, and specifically to the use of open-irrigation ablation catheters, the interference from the irrigated saline at the catheter/tissue interface caused the monitoring of microbubbles with ICE to be quite challenging. Fortunately, it can be argued that the monitoring for tissue overheating at the catheter/tissue interface (i.e., atrial endocardium) during the use of open-irrigation ablation catheters is no longer relevant. Cryoablation using a "point-by-point" approach as with current RF technologies has been associated with disappointing efficacy and very prolonged procedural times due to the requirement of several minutes duration for each ablation lesion delivery. However, there is renewed interest in this technology due to concerns for esophageal injury during application of RF energy at the posterior LA overlying the esophagus, as cryothermy is considered to be less likely to damage the esophagus [14–16]. Some centers have adopted the use of cryoablation for use as an adjunct to RF ablation procedures to be employed over regions of the LA overlying the esophagus to lessen the chance of damage to the esophagus and prevent subsequent development of atrioesophageal fistula.

New tools and techniques to perform PV isolation

There has been development of new technologies to assist the operator with PVI for AF catheter ablation. Some of these technologies have been developed specifically for PVI, whereas other technologies can also be employed for catheter ablation at other sites, such as with electrogram-based ablation, delivery of lines of lesions, targeting of autonomic ganglia, or ablation of non-PV foci.

Various balloon-based technologies have been under investigation, generally designed specifically to deliver arcs or circumferential lesions at the PVs [17]. Such technologies have included the use of cryothermy [18–20] laser [21,22], ultrasound [23–35], and RF energy [26–28]. Typically these technologies have employed a noncompliant balloon and have suffered from inability to isolate the PVs proximally, particularly at the antrum, but instead achieve isolation more distally at the ostium of the PV or even within the PV itself [29,30]. This latter issue has been the "Achilles heel" of such balloon technologies, as the resulting lesion delivery at such a distal location has been associated with lower efficacy by not addressing more proximal sites of triggers, and more troubling also associated with an increase in complications such as PV stenosis and PN damage.

Only a few balloon-based ablation technologies have become available in Europe. To date, the only balloon technology to be approved for use in the United States has been a cryoablation system. Even so, the issues with the nearly obligatory distal location of the delivered ablation lesions still remain. Other balloon-based technologies are under development that would employ a compliant balloon to address these shortcomings [21].

Another new technology has been the development of catheters with various lengths and shapes of the effective ablation delivery region. With use of such catheters, delivery of arcs or lines of lesions might be facilitated. One such system that consists of a "tool kit" of these various technologies has been approved for use in the United States and elsewhere [31,32]. However, additional developments with these types of systems such as irrigation ablation technology would likely facilitate increased adoption of such tools for AF ablation.

Robotic technologies have been developed for use for catheter navigation. Presently, two of such technologies are available [33,34]. One technology utilizes magnetic fields to navigate special magnetic catheters. The magnetic field can be manipulated at a remote workstation to direct the tip of the catheter. The catheter is advanced and retracted with a motor connected to the catheter that is also controlled at the remote workstation. A significant advantage of the magnetic catheter is the physical property of being quite floppy, with virtually no ability to generate excessive contact force against the myocardium to present a risk of perforation. This allows for manipulation of the catheter without or at least with much reduced fluoroscopic guidance. The operator is already at a remote workstation beyond the exposure limits of the fluoroscopic radiation, and the additional decrease in the need for fluoroscopy with the floppy catheter can greatly reduce the radiation exposure to the patient. A major limitation of this robotic technology is the inability to control additional catheters, such as the CMC and/or the ICE catheter. An enhancement to address this issue has been developed and is available in Europe, which is a robotic arm mounted at the bedside to mechanically control the catheter at the remote workstation. However, this technology is not presently available outside of Europe. The use of this magnetic robotic technology for AF catheter ablation has been reported with comparable efficacy and safety to manual techniques [35–37]. One of these reports documented improved safety compared with manual ablation [35].

Another robotic technology that has become available is a system that employs a deflectable sheath controlled at a remote workstation. This deflectable sheath may then be used with a standard mapping catheter. Initial reports revealed comparable efficacy to manual ablation for AF [38,39]. However, serious complications were reported with early experience in particular, including vascular access site complications and cardiac perforation [40,41]. Reports from centers with extensive experience has demonstrated comparable results to manual methods and reduced fluoroscopy times [42,43]. The primary advantage of this system is the ability to use standard catheters rather than specialized catheters as with the magnetic robotic system. However, this system does not offer the safety of the magnetic catheters with regard to potential for excessive forces to the myocardium, so the risk of perforation remains an issue.

Both of these robotic systems offer the advantage of manipulating catheter(s) from a remote workstation, thereby reducing the fluoroscopic radiation exposure to the operator. Additionally, the time that the operator is required to stand at the bedside wearing protective lead garments is greatly reduced, thereby reducing the potential adverse orthopedic effects of such equipment, particularly that of the neck and spine. Such robotic systems offer the potential for navigating catheters with more precision than with a manual technique.

Electrogram-based ablation or CFAE ablation

In addition to PVI and linear lesions, different patterns of electrograms have been targeted during RFCA of AF [44–53] (Table 3.2). These electrograms include areas displaying a greater percentage of continuous activity, temporal activation gradient, fractionation during AF from sites harboring autonomic ganglion, and CFAEs. CFAEs have been most widely studied and form the basis of this section. Intraoperative mapping of AF has shown that CFAEs are found mostly in areas of slow conduction or at points where the wavelets turn around at the end of arcs of functional block. Such CFAEs have relatively short cycle lengths and heterogeneous spatial and temporal distribution. Recent studies have attempted to target these CFAEs in order to terminate and prevent recurrence of AF [44,45,50–52].

In a recent study of 121 patients with AF by Nademanee et al. (57 paroxysmal), CARTO mapping of both atria was performed during spontaneous or induced AF. CFAEs were identified using bipolar recordings filtered at 30–500 Hz and defined by the presence of voltage ≤ 0.15 mV. The definition of CFAE included (1) atrial electrograms that had fractionated electrograms composed of two deflections or more, and/or perturbations of the baseline with continuous deflections of a prolonged activation complex over a 10-second recording period, and (2) atrial electrograms with very short cycle lengths (≤ 120 ms) averaged over a 10-second recording period.

RFA of the area with CFAE was performed in an attempt to eliminate the CFAE. Based on CARTO maps, a biatrial replica was divided into nine separate areas: the septum, including the Bachman bundle; the left posteroseptal mitral annulus and CS ostium; the PVs; the LA roof; the mitral annulus; the cavotricuspid isthmus; the crista terminalis; the right and LAAs; and the SVC–RA junction. Classification and regional distribution of the CFAE is depicted in (Table 3.3). CFAEs were found in seven of the nine regions of both atria, but were mainly confined to the IAS, the PVs, the LA roof, the left posteroseptal mitral annulus, and the CS ostium. The fibrillation cycle length along both sides of the septum was ≤ 120 ms, in contrast with the 235–280 ms length at the left and RAA. According to this report, 92 (76%) of the 121 patients were free of arrhythmia at 1-year follow-up.

However, other studies have shown some improvement or no improvement when ablation of CFAE alone or in combination with PVI is performed, especially in patients with long-standing persistent AF [52] (Figure 3.6, Table 3.4). Another study suggested that CFAE during AF can demonstrate dynamic changes, with some CFAEs having passing activation [45]. In this study, AF was induced in 20 patients with paroxysmal AF. The AF was mapped at 10 different sites in the LA and RA using a high-density multielectrode catheter. Longer electrogram duration was recorded in the LA compared with the RA

Table 3.2 Outcomes of different ablation techniques in chronic AF.

Study name	Year	Number of patients	Follow-up (mo)	Technique	PVI verified	Linear lesions	CFAE	Success rate
Willems et al. Eur Heart J. 2006; 27:2871–2878.	2006	62	14–17	PVI	Yes	Yes	No	45% (63% with linear lesions)
Haïssaguerre et al. J Cardiovasc Electrophysiol. 2000; 11:2–10.	2000	15	11±8	PVI	Yes	No	No	60%
Haïssaguerre et al. J Cardiovasc Electrophysiol. 2005; 16:1138–1147.	2005	60	11±6	PVI	Yes	Yes	Yes	95%
Oral et al. Heart Rhythm. 2005; 2:1165–1172.	2005	80	9±4	CPVA	No	Yes	No	68%
Oral et al. N Engl J Med. 2006; 354:934–941.	2006	146	12	CPVA	No	Yes	No	74%
Ouyang et al. Circulation. 2005; 112:3038–3048.	2005	40	8±2	PVI	Yes	No	No	95%
Kanagaratnam et al. Pacing Clin Electrophysiol. 2001; 24:1774–1779.	2001	71	29±8	PVI	Yes (31%)	No	No	21%
Calo et al. J Am Coll Cardiol. 2006; 47:2504–2512.	2006	80	14±5	CPVA	No	MI	No	72% (85% with biatrial ablation)
Bertaglia et al. Pacing Clin Electrophysiol. 2006; 29:153–158.	2006	74	20±6	CPVA	No	MI	No	70%
Elayi et al. Heart Rhythm. 2008; 5:1658–1664.	2008	144	16	PVAI	Yes	No	Yes	61%

Table 3.3 Classification and regional differences of CFAE distributions.

AF classification	Number of patients (types)	Number of patients at various locations of CFAE distribution
Type I AF: CFAEs localize in only one area	23 (16 PAF and 7 CAF)	10 PVs (4 RSPV, 3 LSPV, 1 LIPV, 2 both RSPV, and LSPV) 8 interatrial septum 4 proximal CS 1 inferolateral aspect of the RA
Types II AF: CFAEs localize in two areas	43 (21 PAF and 22 CAF)	19 PVs and septum 9 septum and proximal CS 4 PVs and left posteroseptal mitral annulus 3 PVand cavotricuspid isthmus 5 septum and mitral annulus 3 septum and the roof of the LA
Type III AF: CFAE localize in ≥3areas	55 (20 PAF and 35 CAF)	46 interatrial septum (83%) 37 PVs (67%) 34 left atrial roof (61%) 32 proximal CS and its ostium (59%) 13 MA (24%) 17 cavotriscuspid isthmus (31%) 4 inferolateral aspect of the RA (7%) 2 SVC and right atrial junction (4%)

Source: Reproduced from Nademanee, McKenzie, Kosar, et al. A new approach for catheter ablation of atrial fibrillation: Mapping of the electrophysiologic substrate. J Am Coll Cardiol 2004; 43:2044–2053.

$(118 \pm 21$ ms vs. 104 ± 23 ms, $p = .001)$. AF cycle length significantly shortened before the occurrence of CFAE compared with baseline in the LA $(174 \pm 32$ ms vs. 186 ± 32 ms, $p = .0001)$ and RA $(177 \pm 31$ ms vs. 188 ± 31 ms, $p = .0001)$, and returned to baseline afterward. A nearly simultaneous activation in all splines was seen in 84% of the recordings, indicating passive activation. This could be due to previously described observations that AF-induced electrogram fractionation was the result of increased variability in propagation velocity and direction of waves emanating from AF sources. However, given the fact that reentrant wavelets are expected to meander, it may not be surprising that, in some cases, location of CFAE could be fleeting in nature.

A hybrid approach combining CFAE with other techniques is usually used in patients undergoing AF ablation. Automated algorithms with CFAE (and other relevant electrograms) and further randomized studies using standard ablation techniques with or without CFAE ablation are needed to understand the role of these complex electrograms in successful ablation of patients with AF.

Linear lesions

Linear lesions were used initially intraoperatively with the aim of preventing the multiple reentrant wavelets that sustain AF. It is not surprising that

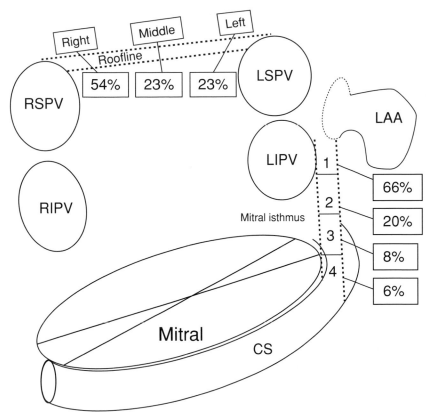

Figure 3.6 Ablation strategy includes isolation at the ostium of the PVs, linear lesion on the roof connecting the upper PVs, and isthmus line along the mitral annulus. This strategy differs from circumferential PV ablation because isolation is confirmed by circular mapping and conduction block along the linear lesion is validated. (Reproduced from Rostock T, O'Neill M, Sanders P, et al. Charaterization of conduction recovery across left atrial linear lesions in patients with paroxysmal and persistent AF. J Cardiovasc Electrophysiol 2006; 17:1106–1111.)

catheter-based ablation procedures pursued a similar strategy. The goal of linear lesions is the achievement of bidirectional conduction block. Despite the use of irrigated tip ablation catheters with 3D anatomical guidance, lesion creation remains challenging [54]. Although a number of linear ablation catheters have been developed over the years [55], few are commercially

Table 3.4 Different ablation approaches in patients with persistent AF using CFAE.

Authors	Number of patients	AF termination	Long-term success	Ablation technique
Oral et al.	50	34% with ibutilide	60%	CFAE + PVI
Verma et al.	40	NA	82%	PVI + CFAE
Oketani et al.	410	80% with ibutilide	81%	CFAE alone

available and thus linear lesions continue to be created with tip ablation catheters at most centers.

Linear lesions have been reported to be associated with conversion of AF either directly to sinus rhythm or to atrial tachycardia, further demonstrating that such lesions may at least in some patients deeply modify the substrate for AF [56,57]. In many patients with a history of persistent AF, conversion to an atrial macroreentry tachycardia is observed during the ablation process and detailed mapping and linear ablation of such tachycardias may result in return to sinus rhythm without the requirement for electrocardioversion. This is particularly true for the recent approaches combining multiple (step-wise) ablation strategies for AF ablation that can result in transformation of AF into organized atrial tachyarrhythmias [58]. Most of these atrial tachycardias are macroreentrant and require linear lesions to be treated [59]. Such organized tachycardias may be observed during the index procedure or emerge upon follow-up. Although complete linear lesions can terminate such organized tachycardias, the development of a gap in conduction block along such lines has the potential for a proarrhythmic effect and can facilitate sustained reentry [60].

For patients in whom AFL has been previously recorded clinically as well as those in whom right AFL is inducible after PVI, ablation of the right atrial cavotricuspid isthmus [61] may be appropriate but on long-term follow-up may of limited added value beyond PVI alone [62,63]. Ablation of the posterolateral mitral isthmus (to the inferior pole of the left PV antrum) has been widely deployed in patients with persistent AF (Figure 3.5) [56,64,65]. One limitation of the mitral isthmus ablation is that it can require supplemental RF applications in the distal CS with its intrinsic safety concerns before conduction block is achieved. A number of approaches have been proposed to overcome this requirement including balloon occlusion of the CS to reduce the heat sink effect of the CS blood flow during endocardial ablation [66] and modification of the line to a more superolateral trajectory [67].

With wide area circumferential pulmonary antral isolation approach, the distance between the contralateral encirclements is greatly reduced posteriorly. Thus a left atrial roofline (which can be created sufficiently superiorly to minimize ablation adjacent to the esophagus) can be achieved with a short transverse lesion connecting the two encirclements. Following the creation of such a lesion, evidence of an organizational effect can often be seen [65]. However, in some patients, particularly those with long-standing persistent AF, high frequency activity may persist in the posterior left atrial wall. More recently the creation of a second transverse linear lesion between the inferior poles of the contralateral encirclements has been deployed in order to complete a box isolation of the posterior left atrial wall [68]. This latter technique has the advantage of isolating a large of area of high frequency activity where triggers and drivers are more likely to occur than other parts of the atria. With respect to the risk of atrioesophageal fistula, this technique does not necessitate more ablation over the posterior wall than conventional wide area circumferential ablation of the PV antra and has been combined with esophageal cooling [69]. Supplemental linear ablation on the anterior wall of the LA appears to be of lesser potential impact [70].

Autonomic GP ablation

Autonomic influences in the heart are produced by the extrinsic (central) and intrinsic cardiac autonomic nervous systems. The extrinsic cardiac autonomic nervous system is comprised of the vagosympathetic system from the brain and spinal cord to the heart. The intrinsic cardiac autonomic nervous system contains clusters of autonomic ganglia (GP) located in epicardial fat pads on the left and right atria and in the ligament of Marshall [71,72]. The intrinsic nervous system receives the input from the extrinsic system, but acts independently to modulate numerous cardiac functions, including automaticity, contractility, and conduction [73,74]. The GP contain afferent neurons from the atrial myocardium and from the extrinsic autonomic nervous system, efferent cholinergic and adrenergic neurons with heavy innervation of the PV myocardium and the atrial myocardium surrounding the GP), and an interconnecting neurons. The interconnecting neurons create a communication network between the different GP.

GP activation includes both parasympathetic and sympathetic stimulation of the atrium surrounding the GP and the closest PV [71]. Parasympathetic stimulation markedly shortens APD, especially in the PV myocardium. Sympathetic stimulation increases calcium loading and calcium release from the sarcoplasmic reticulum (larger and longer calcium transient). The combination of short APD (early repolarization) and longer calcium release results in early afterrepolarizations and triggered firing, initiating PV firing and AF [75,76].

Localization of left atrial GP by endocardial high-frequency stimulation

In patients with AF, endocardial HFS (cycle length 50 ms, 12-Volt actual output, 10-ms pulse width, using a Grass stimulator coupled to an isolation unit) produces a positive vagal response (transient AV block during AF and hypotension, Figure 3.7), allowing the identification and localization of five major left atrial GP (superior left GP, inferior left GP, Marshall tract GP, anterior right GP, and inferior right GP, Figure 3.8) [77]. High-density electroanatomical maps of the LA and PVs obtained during AF shows that the FAPs are located in four main left atrial areas: LAA ridge FAP area, superior-left FAP area, inferoposterior FAP area, and anterior-right FAP area, Figure 3.8). All five GP are located within one of the four FAP areas (Figure 3.9) [7]. These observations suggest a relationship between GP activation and the occurrence of FAP and communication between GP.

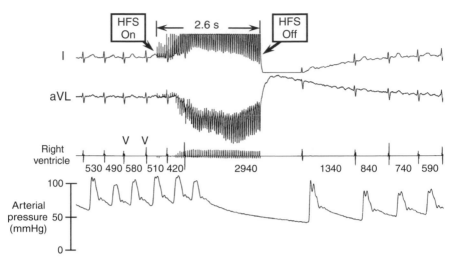

Figure 3.7 Identification of GP using endocardial HFS. The tracings from the top are ECG lead I, aVL, electrograms from the right ventricle, and arterial pressure. Endocardial HFS (cycle length 50 ms, pulse width 10 ms) is delivered in the posterior LA, 2.0–2.5 cm inferior to the ostium of the LIPV, resulting in transient complete AV block and hypotension (vagal response), identifying the inferior left GP.

Catheter ablation of left atrial GP

For endocardial GP ablation, RF energy can be applied to each site exhibiting a positive vagal response to HFS [77–80]. HFS is repeated after each RF application. If a vagal response is still present, RF energy is reapplied until the vagal response is eliminated. Elimination of the vagal response to HFS at each GP generally requires 3–10 RF applications (usually 30–35–40 W for 30–40 seconds but less when close to the esophagus).

In a population of 63 patients with paroxysmal AF undergoing ablation of the left atrial GP ablation followed by PV antrum isolation, GP ablation alone (prior to PV antrum isolation) decreased the occurrence of PV firing from 47 (75%) of 63 patients before GP ablation to only 9 (14%) of the 63 patients ($p < .01$) after GP ablation [77]. PV antrum isolation was then performed, which eliminated PV firing in the remaining 9 patients (0/63 patients), suggesting that PV antrum isolation interrupted axons extending from GP that were not destroyed by the GP ablation procedure (outside the area ablated). The description in earlier studies of the elimination of PV firing by PVI, without targeting the sites of firing [81], may be explained by the interruption of the axons extending from the GP to the PV myocardium.

A similar relationship is present between CFAE ablation [44] and GP ablation. GP ablation alone often eliminates the majority of CFAEs, despite ablating a much smaller area than the overall CFAE area. CFAE ablation may

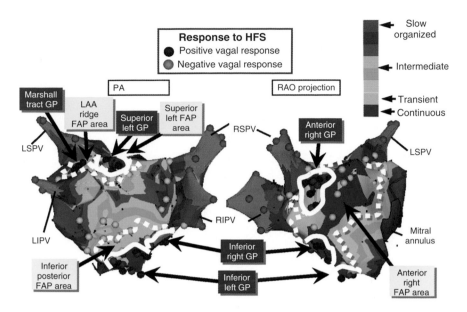

Figure 3.8 Relationship between locations of FAP and GP in patients undergoing catheter ablation of AF. An electroanatomical map of FAP in a patient with paroxysmal AF. Electrograms were recorded for 2.5 seconds at each site. Sites exhibiting FAP for the entire 2.5 seconds were classified as "Continuous FAP" and colored red. Sites with FAP for ≥0.5 second, but organized atrial potentials for the remainder of the 2.5 seconds, were classified as "Transient FAP" and colored orange. Sites exhibiting periods of irregular morphology and cycle length, but not very rapid, were classified as "Intermediate FAP" and colored green-light-blue. Sites exhibiting large amplitude and discrete atrial potentials with average cycle length ≥ 180 ms were classified as "Slow Organized" atrial potentials and colored purple. A FAP *area* was defined as a contiguous area of FAP (Continuous or Transient FAP). Four FAP areas were identified: LAA ridge FAP area, superior left FAP area, inferior posterior FAP area, and anterior right FAP area. Sites where endocardial HFS produced a vagal response (shown in Figure 3.1) are marked by brown tags, corresponding the five major GP areas: (1) Marshall tract GP; (2) superior left GP; (3) inferior left GP; (4) inferior right GP; and (5) anterior right GP. HFS failed to produce a vagal response at the sites marked by orange tags.

eliminate much of the fractionation by ablating the axons without ablation of the GP cell bodies, which may be less likely to be permanent.

GP ablation also decreased the inducibility of sustained AF (>3 minutes duration) from 43 (68%) of 63 patients to 23 (37%) of 63 patients ($p < .01$). The addition of PV antrum isolation further decreased the inducibility of sustained AF to 11 (17%) of 63 patients ($p < .01$) [77,78,80]. FAP mapping of the LA and four PVs was obtained before and after GP ablation (prior to PV antrum isolation) in five patients in whom sustained AF continued after GP ablation. Although ablation sites were limited to sites of positive vagal response to HRS, GP ablation markedly reduced the area of FAP (median 26.9 cm^2 to 2.3 cm^2, $p < .01$) in all five patients [77].

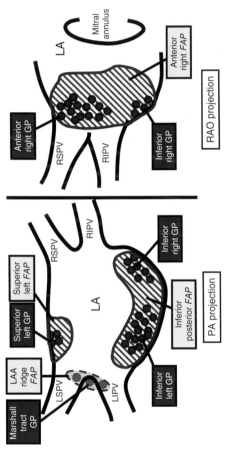

Figure 3.9 Schematic representation of the correlation between the FAP areas and GP locations. Brawn tags indicate sites with a positive HFS response, identifying five major GP areas. Red crossed-hatch areas indicate FAP areas. All five GP are located within one of the four FAP areas.

Ablation of AF nests guided by real-time spectral mapping in sinus rhythm

Pachon et al. have developed a system for real-time spectral mapping using FFT in sinus rhythm [82]. This mapping strategy identifies sites in which the unfiltered, bipolar atrial electrograms contain unusually high frequencies, namely, fibrillar myocardium or the so-called AF Nest (Figure 3.10). The investigators successfully targeted biatrial AF Nests, without intentional PVI, as a novel approach for AF ablation.

Oh et al. compared CFAE sites and AF Nests in an animal model of vagally mediated AF and concluded that these sites did not share identical anatomical locations [83].

In an attempt to further modify the AF substrate and to improve long-term ablation success, Arruda et al. evaluated the adjunctive role of AF Nest ablation to antral PVI and SVC isolation in a prospective randomized study at the Cleveland Clinic [84]. Typically for AF Nest ablation, RF delivery for 20–30 seconds abolishes the high-frequency potentials normalizing the spectrum.

Importantly, full lesion thickness or linear lesions are not required; therefore, this approach is less likely to create a substrate for macroreentrant atrial tachyarrhythmias while sparing viable atrial myocardium. The adjunct of AF Nest ablation resulted in a 10% decrease of recurrence as compared to conventional antral PVI and SVC isolation [85].

Sequential ablation strategy

A stepwise approach has been recently developed in patients with long-lasting persistent AF with different sequences that target multiple atrial areas [86]. The endpoint of the sequential ablation strategy is termination of AF. This can be achieved by passing directly from AF either to sinus rhythm or, more commonly, to atrial tachycardia, which is then mapped and ablated. The first step consists in PVI using antral isolation. As only 12% of AF will stop at that stage, the second step is frequently needed. It requires ECG-guided ablation targeting continuous electrical activities, focal sources, areas with temporal gradient, etc. The last step uses linear lesions and is used in case of persisting AF/AT after the first two steps. The mitral isthmus line is deployed after the roofline as a last resort given the difficulties observed in achieving a complete block.

Once sinus rhythm has been restored, PVI and linear lesions are checked for completeness and areas reablated if needed. It should be emphasized that this approach represents an extensive procedure associated with significant risks and requires careful and individualized risk–benefit assessment. However, it is associated with unprecedented success rate in long-standing AF, particularly when AF termination is achieved during the index procedure. The optimal timing for ablation is before 23 months of uninterrupted AF, and when the LA parasternal diameter (echographically measured) is <50 mm.

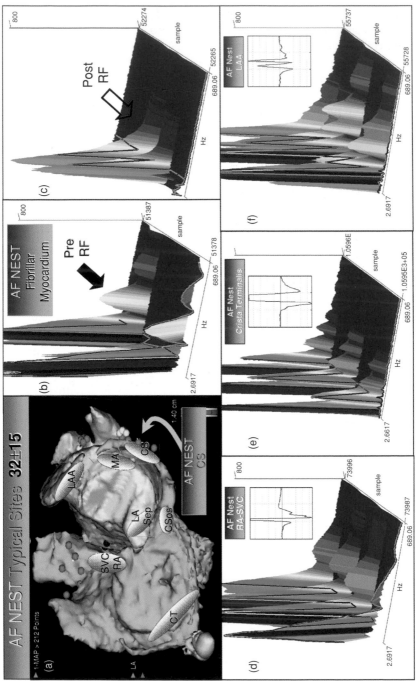

Figure 3.10 (a) The typical locations exhibiting fibrillar myocardium (AF Nest) during real-time spectral mapping in sinus rhythm, following PVI, are shown in a segmented 3D contrast cardiac CT of a patient presenting for AF ablation. Note in (b), the frequency spectra of two consecutive bipolar atrial electrograms (AF Nest) recorded from the CS (arrow in (a)). RF delivery up to 35 W for 20 seconds eliminated the fibrillar pattern shown in (c). Additional examples of AF Nests recorded from other regions are shown in (d)–(f).

Future technologies

In order to improve permanent transmural lesion formation, contact force sensing technology (Biosense Webster and Endosense SA) is currently under clinical investigation. The contact force sensor integrates within the distal tip of a conventional mapping and ablation catheter, providing real-time catheter tip-to-tissue contact feedback. Preliminary results using the Endosense catheter demonstrate feasibility in using this new technology for PVI. Several ongoing studies will determine whether the addition of contact force measurement during AF ablation will result in safer and improved procedural outcome. An alternative means of contact force assessment utilizes local impedance changes between catheter tip and cardiac tissue. The software integrates with the Ensite NavX electroanatomical mapping system and initial animal and human studies have shown its clinical utility during mapping and ablation within the LA [87,88].

The ability to register real-time in-tissue temperature during ablation could potentially facilitate better lesion formation. Using microwave radiometry, very early in-human data demonstrate a correlation between in-tissue temperature and lesion transmurality. Future studies are needed to assess the system's feasibility during AF ablation.

The remote magnetic mapping and ablation system by Magnetecs promises real-time catheter maneuverability within a magnetic field of 1.5 T. The system uses eight electrical magnets that can be switched off. Hence, no magnetic shielding of the examination room is needed. The only system in investigational use is located at La Paz Hospital in Madrid, Spain, and currently studies are underway to test the system's mapping capabilities within humans.

The Amigo robotic arm by Catheter Robotics can be mounted on any conventional examination table and facilitate remote-controlled movement of mapping and ablation catheters. The system is available in Europe and can be integrated with any electroanatomical mapping system. Clinical data are limited with one trial currently recruiting patients to assess the system's ability to navigate and map within the human heart.

A new electroanatomical mapping system is currently being developed that uses a basket-shaped mapping catheter to facilitate acquisition of several thousand mapping points within several minutes. Initial clinical data indicate that the system is able to map complex left atrial arrhythmias in humans.

References

1. Haïssaguerre M, Jaïs P, Shah DC, et al. Spontaneous initiation of atrial fibrillation by ectopic beats originating in the pulmonary veins. N Engl J Med 1998; 339:659–666.
2. Haïssaguerre M, Shah DC, Jaïs P, et al. Electrophysiological breakthroughs from the left atrium to the pulmonary veins. Circulation 2000; 102:2463–2465.
3. Pappone C, Oreto G, Rosanio S, et al. Atrial electroanatomic remodeling after circumferential radiofrequency pulmonary vein ablation: Efficacy of an anatomic approach in a large cohort of patients with atrial fibrillation. Circulation 2001; 104:2539–2544.

4. Pappone C, Rosanio S, Oreto G, Tocchi M, et al. Circumferential radiofrequency ablation of pulmonary vein ostia: A new anatomic approach for curing atrial fibrillation. Circulation 2000; 102:2619–2628.

5. Pappone C, Manguso F, Vicedomini G, et al. Prevention of iatrogenic atrial tachycardia after ablation of atrial fibrillation: A prospective randomized study comparing circumferential pulmonary vein ablation with a modified approach. Circulation 2004; 110:3036–3042.

6. Pappone C, Santinelli V, Manguso F, et al. Pulmonary vein denervation enhances long-term benefit after circumferential ablation for paroxysmal atrial fibrillation. Circulation 2004; 109:327–334.

7. Saad EB, Rossillo A, Saad CP, et al. Pulmonary vein stenosis after radiofrequency ablation of atrial fibrillation: Functional characterization, evolution, and influence of the ablation strategy. Circulation 2003; 108:3102–3107.

8. Ouyang F, Bansch D, Ernst S, et al. Complete isolation of left atrium surrounding the pulmonary veins: New insights from the double-Lasso technique in paroxysmal atrial fibrillation. Circulation 2004; 110:2090–2096.

9. Verma A, Marrouche NF, Natale A. Pulmonary vein antrum isolation: Intracardiac echocardiography-guided technique. J Cardiovasc Electrophysiol 2004; 15:1335–1340.

10. Di Biase L, Elayi CS, Fahmy TS, et al. Atrial fibrillation ablation strategies for paroxysmal patients: Randomized comparison between different techniques. Circ Arrhythm Electrophysiol 2009; 2:113–119.

11. Elayi CS, Verma A, Di Biase L, et al. Ablation for longstanding permanent atrial fibrillation: Results from a randomized study comparing three different strategies. Heart Rhythm 2008; 5:1658–1664.

12. Marrouche NF, Martin DO, Wazni O, et al. Phased-array intracardiac echocardiography monitoring during pulmonary vein isolation in patients with atrial fibrillation: Impact on outcome and complications. Circulation 2003; 107:2710–2716.

13. Wood MA, Shaffer KM, Ellenbogen AL, Ownby ED. Microbubbles during radiofrequency catheter ablation: Composition and formation. Heart Rhythm 2005; 2:397–403.

14. Ahmed H, Neuzil P, d'Avila A, et al. The esophageal effects of cryoenergy during cryoablation for atrial fibrillation. Heart Rhythm 2009; 6:962–969.

15. Herweg B, Ali R, Khan N, Ilercil A, Barold SS. Esophageal contour changes during cryoablation of atrial fibrillation. Pacing Clin Electrophysiol 2009; 32:711–716.

16. Ripley KL, Gage AA, Olsen DB, Van Vleet JF, Lau CP, Tse HF. Time course of esophageal lesions after catheter ablation with cryothermal and radiofrequency ablation: Implication for atrio-esophageal fistula formation after catheter ablation for atrial fibrillation. J Cardiovasc Electrophysiol 2007; 18:642–646.

17. Schmidt B, Chun KR, Metzner A, Ouyang F, Kuck KH. Balloon catheters for pulmonary vein isolation. Herz 2008; 33:580–584.

18. Ahmed H, Neuzil P, Skoda J, et al. The permanency of pulmonary vein isolation using a balloon cryoablation catheter. J Cardiovasc Electrophysiol 2010; 21:731–737.

19. Klein G, Oswald H, Gardiwal A, et al. Efficacy of pulmonary vein isolation by cryoballoon ablation in patients with paroxysmal atrial fibrillation. Heart Rhythm 2008; 5:802–806.

20. Neumann T, Vogt J, Schumacher B, et al. Circumferential pulmonary vein isolation with the cryoballoon technique results from a prospective 3-center study. J Am Coll Cardiol 2008; 52:273–278.

21. Dukkipati SR, Neuzil P, Skoda J, et al. Visual balloon-guided point-by-point ablation: Reliable, reproducible, and persistent pulmonary vein isolation. Circ Arrhythm Electrophysiol 2010; 3:266–273.

22. Reddy VY, Neuzil P, Themistoclakis S, et al. Visually-guided balloon catheter ablation of atrial fibrillation: Experimental feasibility and first-in-human multicenter clinical outcome. Circulation 2009; 120:12–20.

23. Metzner A, Chun KR, Neven K, et al. Long-term clinical outcome following pulmonary vein isolation with high-intensity focused ultrasound balloon catheters in patients with paroxysmal atrial fibrillation. Europace 2010; 12:188–193.

24. Natale A, Pisano E, Shewchik J, et al. First human experience with pulmonary vein isolation using a through-the-balloon circumferential ultrasound ablation system for recurrent atrial fibrillation. Circulation 2000; 102:1879–1882.

25. Schmidt B, Chun KR, Metzner A, Fuernkranz A, Ouyang F, Kuck KH. Pulmonary vein isolation with high-intensity focused ultrasound: Results from the HIFU 12F study. Europace 2009; 11:1281–1288.

26. Arruda MS, He DS, Friedman P, et al. A novel mesh electrode catheter for mapping and radiofrequency delivery at the left atrium-pulmonary vein junction: A single-catheter approach to pulmonary vein antrum isolation. J Cardiovasc Electrophysiol 2007; 18:206–211.

27. Mansour M, Forleo GB, Pappalardo A, et al. Initial experience with the Mesh catheter for pulmonary vein isolation in patients with paroxysmal atrial fibrillation. Heart Rhythm 2008; 5:1510–1516.

28. Neumann T, Kuniss M, Erkapic D, et al. Acute and long-term results of PVI at antrum using a novel high-density mapping catheter without help of 3D electro-anatomic mapping in patients with paroxysmal and chronic atrial fibrillation. J Interv Card Electrophysiol 2010; 27:101–108.

29. Phillips KP, Schweikert RA, Saliba WI, et al. Anatomic location of pulmonary vein electrical disconnection with balloon-based catheter ablation. J Cardiovasc Electrophysiol 2008; 19:14–18.

30. Reddy VY, Neuzil P, d'Avila A, et al. Balloon catheter ablation to treat paroxysmal atrial fibrillation: What is the level of pulmonary venous isolation? Heart Rhythm 2008; 5:353–360.

31. Boersma LV, Wijffels MC, Oral H, Wever EF, Morady F. Pulmonary vein isolation by duty-cycled bipolar and unipolar radiofrequency energy with a multielectrode ablation catheter. Heart Rhythm 2008; 5:1635–1642.

32. Scharf C, Boersma L, Davies W, et al. Ablation of persistent atrial fibrillation using multielectrode catheters and duty-cycled radiofrequency energy. J Am Coll Cardiol 2009; 54:1450–1456.

33. Ernst S. Magnetic and robotic navigation for catheter ablation: "joystick ablation". J Interv Card Electrophysiol 2008; 23:41–44.

34. Schmidt B, Chun KR, Tilz RR, Koektuerk B, Ouyang F, Kuck KH. Remote navigation systems in electrophysiology. Europace 2008; 10:iii57–61.

35. Bauernfeind T, Akca F, Schwagten B, et al. The magnetic navigation system allows safety and high efficacy for ablation of arrhythmias. Europace 2011; 13:1015–1021.

36. Chun KR, Wissner E, Koektuerk B, et al. Remote-controlled magnetic pulmonary vein isolation using a new irrigated-tip catheter in patients with atrial fibrillation. Circ Arrhythm Electrophysiol 2010; 3:458–464.

37. Katsiyiannis WT, Melby DP, Matelski JL, Ervin VL, Laverence KL, Gornick CC. Feasibility and safety of remote-controlled magnetic navigation for ablation of atrial fibrillation. Am J Cardiol 2008; 102:1674–1676.

38. Saliba W, Reddy VY, Wazni O, et al. Atrial fibrillation ablation using a robotic catheter remote control system: Initial human experience and long-term follow-up results. J Am Coll Cardiol 2008; 51:2407–2411.

39. Schmidt B, Tilz RR, Neven K, Julian Chun KR, Furnkranz A, Ouyang F. Remote robotic navigation and electroanatomical mapping for ablation of atrial fibrillation: Considerations for navigation and impact on procedural outcome. Circ Arrhythm Electrophysiol 2009; 2:120–128.

40. Di Biase L, Natale A, Barrett C, et al. Relationship between catheter forces, lesion characteristics, "popping," and char formation: Experience with robotic navigation system. J Cardiovasc Electrophysiol 2009; 20:436–440.

41. Wazni OM, Barrett C, Martin DO, et al. Experience with the hansen robotic system for atrial fibrillation ablation–lessons learned and techniques modified: Hansen in the real world. J Cardiovasc Electrophysiol 2009; 20:1193–1196.

42. Di Biase L, Wang Y, Horton R, et al. Ablation of atrial fibrillation utilizing robotic catheter navigation in comparison to manual navigation and ablation: Single-center experience. J Cardiovasc Electrophysiol 2009; 20:1328–1335.

43. Hlivak P, Mlcochova H, Peichl P, Cihak R, Wichterle D, Kautzner J. Robotic navigation in catheter ablation for paroxysmal atrial fibrillation: Midterm efficacy and predictors of postablation arrhythmia recurrences. J Cardiovasc Electrophysiol 2011; 22:534–540.

44. Nademanee K, McKenzie J, Kosar E, et al. A new approach for catheter ablation of atrial fibrillation: Mapping of the electrophysiologic substrate. J Am Coll Cardiol 2004; 43:2044–2053.

45. Rostock T, Rotter M, Sanders P, et al. High-density activation mapping of fractionated electrograms in the atria of patients with paroxysmal atrial fibrillation. Heart Rhythm 2006; 3:27–34.

46. Po SS, Scherlag BJ, Yamanashi WS, et al. Experimental model for paroxysmal atrial fibrillation arising at the pulmonary vein-atrial junctions. Heart Rhythm 2006; 3:201–208.

47. Lemery R, Birnie D, Tang AS, Green M, Gollob M. Feasibility study of endocardial mapping of ganglionated plexuses during catheter ablation of atrial fibrillation. Heart Rhythm 2006; 3:387–396.

48. Tan AY, Li H, Wachsmann-Hogiu S, Chen LS, Chen PS, Fishbein MC. Autonomic innervation and segmental muscular disconnections at the human pulmonary vein-atrial junction: Implications for catheter ablation of atrial-pulmonary vein junction. J Am Coll Cardiol 2006; 48:132–143.

49. Scanavacca M, Pisani CF, Hachul D, et al. Selective atrial vagal denervation guided by evoked vagal reflex to treat patients with paroxysmal atrial fibrillation. Circulation 2006; 114:876–885.

50. Verma A, Patel D, Famey T, et al. Efficacy of adjuvant anterior left atrial ablation during intracardiac echocardiography-guided pulmonary vein antrum isolation for atrial fibrillation. J Cardiovasc Electrophysiol 2007; 18:151–156.

51. Oketani N, Lockwood E, Nademanee K. Incidence and mode of AF termination during substrate ablation of AF guided solely by complex fractionated atrial electrogram mapping (abstract). Circulation 2008; 118:S925.

52. Oral H, Chugh A, Yoshida K, et al. A randomized assessment of the incremental role of ablation of complex fractionated atrial electrograms after antral pulmonary vein isolation for long-lasting persistent atrial fibrillation. J Am Coll Cardiol 2009; 53:782–789.

53. Takahashi Y, O'Neill M, Hocini M, et al. Characterization of electrograms associated with termination of chronic atrial fibrillation by catheter ablation. J Am Coll Cardiol 2008; 51:1003–1010.

54. Lavergne T, Jaïs P, Haïssaguerre M, et al. Evaluation of a single passage RF ablation line in animal atria using an irrigated tip catheter. Circulation 1997; 96:259-I.

55. Keane D, Hynes B, Lamkin R, et al. Linear radiofrequency microcatheter ablation guided by phased array intracardiac echocardiography combined with temperature decay. PACE 2009; 32:1543–1552.

56. Kottkamp H, Hindricks G, Autschbach R, et al. Specific linear left atrial lesions in atrial fibrillation: Intraoperative radiofrequency ablation using minimally invasive surgical techniques. J Am Coll Cardiol 2002; 40:475–480.

57. Jaïs P, Shah DC, Haïssaguerre M, et al. Efficacy and safety of septal and left-atrial linear ablation for atrial fibrillation. Am J Cardiol 1999; 84:139R–146R.

58. Knecht S, Hocini M, Wright M, et al. Left atrial linear lesions are required for successful treatment of persistent atrial Fibrillation. European Heart Journal 2008; 29:2359–2366.

59. Jaïs P, Shah D, Haïssaguerre M, et al. Mapping and ablation of left atrial flutters. Circulation 2000; 101:2928–2934.

60. Raviele A, Themistoclakis S, Rossillo A, Bonso A. Iatrogenic postatrial fibrillation ablation left atrial tachycardia/flutter: How to prevent and treat it? J Cardiovasc Electrophysiol 2005; 16:298–301.

61. Scharf C, Veerareddy S, Ozaydin M, et al. Clinical significance of inducible atrial flutter during pulmonary vein isolation in patients with atrial fibrillation. J Am Coll Cardiol 2004; 43:2057–2062.

62. Wazni O, Marrouche N, Martin D, et al. Randomized study comparing combined pulmonary vein-left atrial junction disconnection and cavotricuspid isthmus ablation versus pulmonary vein-left atrial junction disconnection alone in patients presenting with typical atrial flutter and atrial fibrillation. Circulation 2003; 108:2479.

63. Schmidt M, Daccarett M, Segerson N, et al. Atrial flutter ablation in inducible patients during pulmonary vein atrum isolation: A randomized comparison. PACE 2008; 31:1592–1597.

64. Jaïs P, Hsu LF, Rotter M, et al. Mitral isthmus ablation for atrial fibrillation. J Cardiovasc Electrophysiol 2005; 16:1157–1159.

65. Hocini M, Jaıs P, Sanders P, et al. Techniques, evaluation, and consequences of linear block at the left atrial roof in paroxysmal atrial fibrillation: A prospective randomized study. Circulation 2005; 112:3688–3696.

66. Reddy VY, Ruskin JN, D'Avila A. Balloon occlusion of the coronary sinus to facilitate mitral isthmus ablation. J Cardiovasc Electrophysiol 2008; 19:651.

67. Schmidt, Ouyang, Kuck, et al. Superolateral mitral isthmus ablation. AHA 2009; Circulation supplement.

68. Kumagai K, Nakashima H. Noncontact mapping-guided catheter ablation of atrial fibrillation. Circ J 2009; 73:233–241.

69. Kumagai K, Muraoka S, Mitsutake C, Takashima H, Nakashima H. A new approach for complete isolation of the posterior left atrium including pulmonary veins for atrial fibrillation. J Cardiovasc Electrophysiol 2007; 18:1047–1052.

70. Verma A, Patel D, Famy T, et al. Efficacy of adjuvant anterior LA ablation during pulmonary vein antrum isolation for AF. J Cardiovasc Electrophysiol 2007; 18:151–156.

71. Armour JA, Yuan BX, Macdonald S, et al. Gross and microscopic anatomy of the human intrinsic cardiac nervous system. Anat Rec 1997; 247:289–298.

72. Pauza DH, Skripka V, Pauziene N, et al. Morphology, distribution, and variability of the epicardiac neural ganglionated subplexuses in the human heart. Anat Rec 2000; 259:353–382.

73. Armour JA, Hageman GR, Randall WC. Arrhythmias induced by local cardiac nerve stimulation. Am J Physiol 1972; 223:1068–1075.

74. Scherlag BJ, Nakagawa H, Jackman WM, et al. Electrical stimulation to identify neural elements on the heart: Their role in atrial fibrillation. J Interventional Electrophysiol 2005; 13:37–42.

75. Patterson E, Po SS, Scherlag BJ, et al. Triggered firing in pulmonary veins initiated by in vitro autonomic nerve stimulation. Heart Rhythm 2005; 2:624–631.

76. Patterson E, Lazzara R, Szabo B, et al. Sodium-calcium exchange initiated by the Ca^{2+} transient: An arrhythmia trigger within pulmonary veins. J Am Coll Cardiol 2006; 47:1196–1206.

77. Nakagawa H, Scherlag BJ, Patterson E, Ikeda A, Lockwood D, Jackman, WM. Pathophysiologic basis of autonomic ganglionated plexi ablation in patients with atrial fibrillation. Heart Rhythm 2009; 6:S26-S34.

78. Nakagawa H, Yokoyama K, Scherlag BJ, et al. Ablation of autonomic ganglia In: Calkins H, Jaïs P, Steinberg JS, eds. A Practical Approach to Catheter Ablation of Atrial Fibrillation. Philadelphia: Wolters Kluwer/Lippincott Williams & Wilkins; 2008, pp. 218–230.

79. Nakagawa H, Scherlag BJ, Lockwood D, et al. Localization of left atrial autonomic ganglionated plexuses using endocardial and epicardial high frequency stimulation in patients with atrial fibrillation. Heart Rhythm 2005; 2:S10. Abstract.

80. Nakagawa H, Scherlag BJ, Wu R, et al. Addition of selective ablation of autonomic ganglia to pulmonary vein atrum isolation for treatment of paroxysmal and persistent atrial fibrillation. Circulation 2004; 110:III-543. Abstract

81. Macle L, Jaïs P, Scavee C, et al. Electrophysiologically guided pulmonary vein isolation during sustained atrial fibrillation. J Cardiovasc Electrophysiol 2003; 14:255–260.

82. Pachon MJ, Pachon ME, Lobo TJ, et al. A new treatment for atrial fibrillation based on spectral analysis to guide the catheter RF-ablation. Europace 2004; 6:590–601.

83. Oh S, Kong H, Choi E, Kim HC, Choi Y. Complex fractionated electrograms and AF nests in vagally mediated atrial fibrillation. Pacing and Clinical Electrophysiology 2010; 33:1497–1503.

84. Arruda M, Prasad SK, Kozeluhova M, et al. Combined spectral mapping guided AF-Nests ablation and pulmonary vein antrum isolation: A new approach to improve AF ablation success. Heart Rhythm 2006; 4:S52.

85. Arruda M, Natale A. Ablation of permanent AF: Adjunctive strategies to pulmonary veins isolation: Targeting AF NEST in sinus rhythm and CFAE in AF. J Interv Card Electrophysiol 2008; 23:51–57.

86. Haïssaguerre M, Sanders P, Hocini M, et al. Catheter ablation of long-lasting persistent atrial fibrillation: Critical structures for termination. J Cardiovasc Electrophysiol 2005; 16:1125–1137.

87. Piorkowski C, Sih H, Sommer P, et al. First in human validation of impedance-based catheter tip-to-tissue contact assessment in the left atrium. J Cardiovasc Electrophysiol 2009; 20:1366–1373.

88. Holmes D, Fish JM, Byrd IA, et al. Contact sensing provides a highly accurate means to titrate radiofrequency ablation lesion depth. J Cardiovasc Electrophysiol 2010; 22:684–690.

89. Oral H, Scharf C, Chugh A, et al. Catheter ablation for paroxysmal atrial fibrillation: segmental pulmonary vein ostial ablation versus left atrial ablation. Circulation 2003; 108:2355–2360.

Endpoints of catheter ablation for atrial fibrillation

Michel Haïssaguerre[1], Conor Barrett[2], Luigi Di Biase[3], Sabine Ernst[4], Fiorenzo Gaita[5], Javier E. Sanchez[3], Prashanthan Sanders[6], Richard J. Schilling[7], Stephan Willems[8]

[1]Cardiology Department, Hôpital Haut-Lévêque, CHU de Bordeaux, Bordeaux, France
[2]Cardiac Arrhythmia Service, Massachusetts General Hospital, Boston, MA, USA
[3]Texas Cardiac Arrhythmia Institute, St. David's Medical Center, Austin, TX, USA
[4]National Heart and Lung Institute, Royal Brompton and Harefield Hospital, Imperial College, London, UK
[5]Internal Medicine Department, University of Turin, Turin, Italy
[6]Centre for Heart Rhythm Disorders, Royal Adelaide Hospital, North Terrace, Adelaide, Australia
[7]Cardiology Department, St. Bartholomew's Hospital, London, UK
[8]Cardiology and Electrophysiology Department, Herzzentrum Hamburg GmbH University, Hamburg, Germany

The goal of catheter ablation is maintenance of SR by means of trigger elimination and substrate modification using the least amount of ablation necessary. Various ablation strategies and targets used in isolation or in combination have been adopted for ablation of AF. A minority of patients (especially young), may have other mechanisms for AF induction (e.g., AVRT/AVNRT inducing AF), and if such mechanism is suspected, the primary target would be the elimination of the initiating arrhythmia. The similarity of published outcomes of these varying strategies is a reflection of the paucity of the data supporting their use and our lack of understanding of AF mechanisms. There are two principles that are, at present, supported by general consensus. First, as the vast majority of triggers for AF originate from the PV, there is an agreement [1] that PVI is an integral part of AF ablation procedure. Second, in some patients (in particular patients with persistent and long-lasting persistent AF), additional substrate modification is required to improve outcomes, although the timing of an expanded ablation strategy is still a matter of debate. However, even these clinically accepted principles have little or conflicting randomized controlled trial data supporting them [2–6].

Atrial Fibrillation Ablation, 2011 Update: The State of the Art based on the VeniceChart International Consensus Document, First Edition. Edited by Andrea Natale and Antonio Raviele.
© 2011 John Wiley & Sons, Ltd. Published 2011 by John Wiley & Sons, Ltd.

The principal procedural endpoints used for catheter ablation of AF depend on the type of AF being treated. Endpoints include completion of a predetermined lesion set [7], termination of AF during ablation [8], and noninducibility of AF following ablation [9,10]. Again, lack of consistent data means that there is still debate surrounding the predictive value of endpoints such as AF termination or noninducibility as endpoints for the procedure.

In patients with paroxysmal AF, it is possible that the termination of AF during ablation is coincidental, although the experience of most operators is that it is unusual for truly paroxysmal AF to persist after PVI. Thus, AF termination during PVI, especially when the vein(s) display more rapid cycles than the LA or while the vein itself remains in fibrillation or tachycardia, likely represents exclusion of an arrhythmogenic ("culprit") vein for that particular patient. In patients with paroxysmal AF, noninducibility seems to be associated with an improved outcome [10,11] during the follow-up. However, there is no current consensus on the definition of noninducibility and the standardization of the induction protocol used. Furthermore, it is likely that the noninducibility of AF might identify a subgroup of patients who have less severe atrial disease (no atrial "vulnerability") and, therefore, are more likely to have a successful outcome. Finally, while noninducibility predicts a better outcome, a proportion of patients who remain inducible at the time of the procedure have a good clinical outcome. For patients with persistent and long-lasting persistent AF, the procedural endpoint is also not standardized. Although restoration of SR by ablation, without the use of AADs or DC cardioversion, appears to be an intuitively ideal endpoint, this is not always achievable and may result in more extensive ablation of tissue that is not associated with AF maintenance. Furthermore, the available data show diverging results in this regard. In some studies, increased procedural success and the modality of recurrence (ATach vs. AF) were associated with restoration to SR by ablation [12,13], but this was not reproduced in other studies [14]. This is probably, at least in part, due to the inhomogeneity with respect to populations (e.g., persistent vs. long-standing persistent AF), differing protocols, and the length of follow-up of patients. Importantly, at this early phase of clinical experience, there have been no randomized comparisons of procedural endpoints to allow definitive conclusions. Until more detailed data are available, completion of a predetermined lesion set incorporating PVI remains the basic procedure and the initial step in the event of repeat ablation [15]. Verification and completion of ablation linear lesion sets are fundamental to minimizing proarrhythmia and arrhythmia recurrence. This includes confirmation of electrical PVI and block across ablated lines. The ablation endpoints of the principal ablation approaches discussed in Chapter 3 are summarized in the following and in Table 4.1.

PV isolation

There is consensus that electrical PVI is the optimal endpoint for ablation targeting the LA–PV junction and is now generally incorporated as the initial

Table 4.1 Endpoints for catheter ablation for AF.

Ablation Technique	Ablation site	Ablation End-Points
Segmental/ostial PVI	PV ostium	Complete elimination or dissociation of PV potentials assessed by a circular catheter
Circumferential PVI	1-2 cm outside PV ostium	Abatement of local bipolar voltage by 90% or <0.05 mV within encircled areas
Antral PVI	PV antrum	Complete elimination of PV potentials with isolation of all PVs and posterior wall assessed by a circular catheter
CFAEs ablation	LA areas where CFAEs recorded	Complete elimination of CFAEs Interruption of AF Non-inducibility of AF
Linear lesions	LA roof and mitral isthmus	Creation and demonstration of line of complete block
Autonomic GP ablation	GP located around PVs	Abolition of vagal reflexes induced by HFS
Nest ablation	Local high frequency activity or focal and centrifugal spread of activation or frequency areas	Abolition of this high sites with temporal gradient between two dipoles
Other structures and thoracic veins	Coronary Sinus, left atrial appendage, Superior vena cava, persistent left superior vena cava, Vein of Marshall	Complete elimination or dissociation of other thoracic vein

lesion set in AF ablation strategies [1,16]. The most objective procedural endpoint is the absence or dissociation of PV potentials recorded from a CMC positioned just inside the PV [17–20]. Sequential RF applications targeting the earliest PV potentials may abolish all PV potentials directly or by means of a subsequent change in activation as secondary breakthroughs are ablated. The same endpoint of electrical PVI is considered optimal for wide-area circumferential PV ablation by many. However, reduction of local bipolar amplitude with low peak-to-peak bipolar potentials (≤ 0.1 mV) inside the encircled area, as well as local endocardial activation time >30 ms between contiguous points lying in the same axial plane on the external and internal side of the line, is still suggested by some authors as a suitable endpoint in order to avoid the necessity for a CMC [21]. Nevertheless, most centers now rely on PVI (as described in the preceding text) as the best endpoint following ablation of the LA–PV junction or antrum. Exit block into the LA can also be proven with pacing maneuvers from inside the PV, but is not considered routine. This is due to lack of evidence supporting its clinical utility and the technical difficulty of ensuring pacing capture of the muscle sleeves inside the vein without far-field capture of the LA or RA.

Outcome after initially successful PVI is still unsatisfactory with respect to success rates of 58% after the initial and 70% after repeat procedures reported in a meta-analysis [22]. Also during long-term follow-up, 1 year after the last ablation procedure for paroxysmal AF, annual recurrence rates remain a persistent problem [23–26]. There are only limited data explaining why this may occur, although one hypothesis is that this may still be due to resumption of PV conduction.

The potential role of intravenous adenosine as an adjunct to increase the rate of permanent PVI has been discussed [27] and is part of an ongoing prospective study (ADVICE). As an additional endpoint, nonexcitability of bilateral circumferential lines following PVI has been introduced [28,29]. In a pilot study, AF recurrences were significantly lower after additional application of RF current until achievement of unexcitability as compared to sole PVI [28]. A larger randomized prospective outcome trial is ongoing.

Electrogram-based ablation or CFAEs ablation

Although the pathophysiologic basis and the standardized definition of CFAE are still controversial, clinical endpoints for ablation have been introduced in this regard: (1) complete elimination of the areas with CFAEs, (2) conversion of AF to normal SR for both paroxysmal AF and persistent/long-lasting persistent AF patients, (3) conversion of AF to an organized atrial tachyarrhythmia (atrial tachycardia or flutter), and (4) noninducibility of AF in paroxysmal AF patients. The role of noninducibility with rapid atrial pacing has not unequivocally been shown to be reliable or necessary endpoint in this setting. Additionally, the local endpoint indicating when the RF should be discontinued is unclear. Thus, currently CFAE ablation is not performed as a primary ablative strategy in the majority of centers. Nevertheless, CFAE ablation is frequently used in case of patients with persistent AF sustaining after PVI during the first [8,12,13] or subsequent procedures [15].

The ablation typically begins at the sites where CFAEs have the shortest local A–A interval. Such sites are unfortunately ubiquitous in persistent AF. It is not known whether ablation of all such sites is necessary or if it is possible to target specific locations and thereby limit the extent of unnecessary ablation and resultant tissue damage and potential complications. Irrespective of electrogram complexity, ablation all along some structures like the CS, LAA [30], and septum may also have an impact on AF perpetuation. Despite demonstration of the potential involvement into the fibrillatory process and increased success rates [30], there is some additional concern with regard to ablation in the LAA. This refers to the potential risk of perforation and LAA disconnection with a subsequently increased likelihood for thrombus formation requiring lifelong anticoagulation.

Importantly, after "defragmentation" and prior ablation (PVI and eventually linear lesions), electrograms may become discrete or organized, allowing a dominant rate (frequency) and specific activation sequence to be identified. In such situations, parameters other than fragmentations may be used.

Local high-frequency activity or focal and centrifugal spread of activation or sites with temporal gradient between two bipoles of conventional mapping catheter (representing local circuit, "rotor" or "AF nest") are potential targets for ablation [31]. Also, following CFAE ablation, AF may "organize" into a macroreentrant arrhythmia, which can be further targeted with linear lesion sets, as discussed in the following.

"Defragmentation" additional to PV isolation has not shown favourable outcome in patients with paroxysmal AF [3,4,5] especially at long term follow-up, although in patients with persistent AF [2,4,5,6] the freedom from recurrence of any atrial tachyarrhythmia even with repeat procedures seems satisfactory. This topic deserves further investigation in ongoing large scale trials. In order to avoid potential complications (e.g. damage to esophagus or circumflex artery) RF application should be carefully monitored and limited when used in areas with adjacent structures prone to RF-induced damage (e.g. 20–30 Watts at the posterior LA, 15–20 watts within coronary sinus) or limiting the RF application to 20–30 secs/site.

Linear lesions

In patients with persistent or long-lasting persistent AF [2–6], the use of adjunctive linear ablation, mainly at the level of LA roof and mitral isthmus, has been associated with higher success rates [10,32,33]. Even after termination of ablation-induced macroreentry tachycardia, the endpoint should be a complete line of linear lesions [34–37] because incomplete lesions are associated with recurrence of atrial arrhythmias [38,39]. Therefore, the electrophysiological endpoint should be demonstration of bidirectional line of block. Conduction block at the LA roof or mitral isthmus can be readily assessed in a manner analogous to that used for the cavotricuspid isthmus—a corridor of double potentials and demonstration of activation moving toward the line of block on both sides (e.g., by means of "differential pacing maneuvres")—which represents an unequivocal endpoint [36]. A complete LA roofline may be demonstrated by activation progressing in a caudal-cranial direction on the posterior wall during left appendage pacing [34]. A complete mitral isthmus line may be demonstrated by an inversion of CS activation sequence from distal–proximal to proximal–distal during pacing from the left appendage [36].

Autonomic GP ablation

Autonomic GP are present in epicardial fat pads and can be identified by high-frequency stimulation. They are often clustered around the PVs. High-frequency stimulation at these sites leads to induction of AF and/or bradycardia or AV block due to increased vagal tone. Abolition of inducible vagal reflexes has been proposed as an endpoint of ablation on the basis of experimental data [40]. It is unclear whether GP should be specifically targeted, given that these sites may be concomitantly ablated in the course of above-described ablation targets. Most centers still do not specifically target such plexi, although these may be affected especially when extended ablation approaches are introduced.

Coronary sinus and other thoracic veins ablation

Similar to triggers arising from the muscle sleeves surrounding the PVs, rapid atrial activity from the musculature of the CS may be a driver for persistent or long-lasting persistent AF. The same electrogram-based approach as discussed in the preceding text can be applied to the CS. Ablation endpoints include organization of CS activity and slowing of local rate. Whether total elimination of CS activity is necessary, remains unclear. Moreover, ablation from within the CS is not infrequently required in order to ensure a line of block across the mitral isthmus line.

Other potential triggers, such as SVC and persistent LS vena cava, can be electrically isolated by ablation technique and endpoints similar to PVI, provided that triggering activity emerging from these structures is demonstrated. Abnormal activity from the vein of Marshall can be eliminated from the opposing LA endocardium and uncommonly requires direct catheterization from within the CS.

Key note.

Primary targets: PVs and/or PV antrum.

Primary goal: Complete electrical isolation of PV.

Careful identification of PV ostia to avoid ablation within the PVs.

Ablation of extra-PV triggers in patients with persistent and long-standing persistent AF (LA roof, mitral isthmus, anterior left septum, CS, LAA). In patients with paroxysmal AF electrical isolation of the PV might be sufficient.

For additional linear lesions, verification of line completeness demonstrated by bidirectional block is of fundamental importance to minimize arrhythmia recurrence.

Ablation of the cavotricuspid isthmus recommended only with history of typical AFL or inducible cavotricuspid isthmus dependent AFL.

No consensus on two endpoints: AF termination during ablation and AF inducibility postablation.

References

1. Calkins H, Brugada J, Packer D, et al. HRS/EHRA/ECAS expert consensus statement on catheter and surgical ablation of atrial fibrillation: Recommendations for personnel, policy, procedures and follow-up. A report of the Heart Rhythm Society (HRS) Task force on Catheter and Surgical Ablation of Atrial Fibrillation developed in partnership with the European Heart Rhythm Society (HRS) Task Force on Catheter and Surgical Ablation of Atrial Fibrillation developed in partnership with the European Heart Rhythm

Association (EHRA) and the European Cardiac Arrhythmia Society (ECAS) in collaboration with the American College of Cardiology (ACC), American Heart Association (AHA), and the Society of Thoracic Surgeons (STS). Endorsed and approved by the governing bodies of the American College of Cardiology, the American Heart Association, the European Heart Rhythm Association, the Society of Thoracic Surgeons, and the Heart Rhythm society. Europace 2007; 9:335–379.

2. Verma A, Mantovan R, Macle L, et al. Substrate and trigger ablation for reduction of atrial fibrillation (STAR AF): A randomized prospective trial. Eur Heart J 2010; 31:1344–1356.

3. Di Biase L, Elayi CS, Fahmy TS, et al. Atrial fibrillation ablation strategies for paroxysmal patients: randomized comparison between different techniques. Circ Arrhythm Electrophysiol 2009; 2:113–119.

4. Li WJ, Bai YY, Zhang HY, et al. Additional ablation of complex fractionated atrial electrograms after pulmonary vein isolation in patients with atrial fibrillation: a meta-analysis. Circ Arrhythm Electrophysiol 2011; 4:143–148.

5. Hayward RM, Upadhyay GA, Mela T, et al. Pulmonary vein isolation with complex fractionated atrial electrogram ablation for paroxysmal and nonparoxysmal atrial fibrillation: A meta-analysis. Heart Rhythm 2011; 8:994–1000.

6. Elayi CS, Verma A, Di Biase L, et al. Ablation for longstanding permanent atrial fibrillation: results from a randomized study comparing three different strategies. Heart Rhythm 2008; 5:1658–1664.

7. Pappone C, Santinelli V. Atrial fibrillation ablation: State of the art. Am J Cardiol 2005; 96:59–64.

8. Haissaguerre M, Sanders P, Hocini M, et al. Catheter ablation of long-lasting persistent atrial fibrillation: Critical structures for termination. J Cardiovasc Electrophysiol 2005; 16:1125–1137.

9. Oral H, Chugh A, Good E, et al. A tailored approach to catheter ablation of paroxysmal atrial fibrillation. Circulation 2006; 113:1824–1831.

10. Jais P, Hocini M, Sanders P, et al. Long-term evaluation of atrial fibrillation ablation guided by noninducibility. Heart Rhythm 2006; 3:140–145.

11. Oral H, Chugh A, Lemola K, et al. Noninducibility of atrial fibrillation as an end point of left atrial circumferential ablation for paroxysmal atrial fibrillation: A randomized study. Circulation 2004; 110:2797–2801.

12. O'Neill MD, Wright M, Knecht S, et al. Long-term follow-up of persistent atrial fibrillation ablation using termination as a procedural endpoint. Eur Heart J 2009; 9:1105–1112.

13. Rostock T, Steven D, Hoffmann B, et al. Chronic atrial fibrillation is a biatrial arrhythmia. Data from catheter ablation of chronic atrial fibrillation aiming arrhythmia termination using a sequential ablation approach. Circ Arrhythmia Electrophysiol 2008; 1:344–353.

14. Elayi CS, Di Biase L, Barrett C, et al. Atrial fibrillation termination as a procedural endpoint during ablation in long-standing persistent atrial fibrillation. Heart Rhythm 2010; 9:1216–1223.

15. Tilz R, Chun KR, Schmidt B, et al. Catheter ablation of long-standing persistent atrial fibrillation: A lesson from circumferential pulmonary vein isolation. J Cardiovasc Electrophysiol 2010; 10:1085–1093.

16. Keane D, Reddy V, Ruskin J. Emerging concepts on catheter ablation of atrial fibrillation from the Tenth Annual Boston Atrial Fibrillation Symposium. J Cardiovasc Electrophysiol 2005; 16:1025–1028.

17. Ouyang F, Bänsch D, Ernst S, et al. Complete isolation of left atrium surrounding the pulmonary veins: New insights from the double-Lasso technique in paroxysmal atrial fibrillation. Circulation 2004; 110:2090–2096.

18. Verma A, Marrouche NF, Natale A. Pulmonary vein antrum isolation: Intracardiac echocardiography-guided technique. J Cardiovasc Electrophysiol 2004; 15:1335–1340.
19. Hocini M, Sanders P, Jais P, et al. Techniques for curative treatment of atrial fibrillation. J Cardiovasc Electrophysiol 2004; 15:1467–1471.
20. Sauer WH, McKernan ML, Lin D, Gerstenfeld EP, Callans DJ, Marchlinski FE. Clinical predictors and outcomes associated with acute return of pulmonary vein conduction during pulmonary vein isolation for treatment of atrial fibrillation. Heart Rhythm 2006; 3:1024–1028.
21. Pappone C, Rosanio S, Oreto G, et al. Circumferential radiofrequency ablation of pulmonary vein ostia: A new anatomic approach for curing atrial fibrillation. Circulation 2000; 102:2619–2628.
22. Calkins H, Reynolds MR, Spector P, et al. Treatment of atrial fibrillation with antiarrhythmic drugs or radiofrequency ablation: Two systematic literature reviews and meta-analysis. Circ Arrhythm Electrophysiol 2009; 2:349–361.
23. Ouyang F, Tilz R, Chun J, et al. Long-term results of catheter ablation in paroxysmal atrial fibrillation: Lessons from a 5-year follow-up. Circulation 2010; 122:2368–2377.
24. Weerasooriya R, Khairy P, Litalien J, et al. Catheter ablation for atrial fibrillation: Are results maintained at 5 years of follow up? J Am Coll Cardiol 2011; 57:160–166.
25. Hunter RJ, Berriman TJ, Diab I, et al. Long-term efficacy of catheter ablation for atrial fibrillation: Impact of additional targeting fractionated electrograms. Heart 2010; 96:1372–1378.
26. Medi C, Sparks PB, Morton JB, et al. Pulmonary vein antral isolation for paroxysmal atrial fibrillation: Results from long-term follow-up. J Cardiovasc Electrophysiol 2011; 22:137–141.
27. Arentz T, Macle L, Kalusche D, et al. 'Dormant' pulmonary vein conduction revealed by adenosine after ostial radiofrequency catheter ablation. J Cardiovasc Electrophysiol 2004; 15:1041–1047.
28. Eitel C, Hindricks G, Sommer P, et al. Circumferential pulmonary vein isolation and linear left atrial ablation as a single-catheter technique to achieve bidirectional conduction block: The pace-and-ablate approach. Heart Rhythm 2010; 7:157–164.
29. Steven D, Reddy VY, Inada K, et al. Loss of pace capture on the ablation line: A new marker for complete radiofrequency lesions to achieve pulmonary vein isolation Heart Rhythm 2010; 7:323–330.
30. Di Biase L, Burkhardt JD, Mohanty P, et al. Left atrial appendage: An underrecognized trigger site of atrial fibrillation. Circulation 2010; 122:109–118.
31. Jais P, O'Neill MD, Takahashi Y, et al. Stepwise catheter ablation of chronic atrial fibrillation: Importance of discrete anatomic sites for termination. J Cardiovasc Electrophysiol 2006; 17:S28–S36.
32. Willems S, Klemm H, Rostock T, et al. Substrate modification combined with pulmonary vein isolation improves outcome of catheter ablation in patients with persistent atrial fibrillation: A prospective randomized comparison. Eur Heart J 2006; 27:2871–2878.
33. Gaita F, Caponi D, Scaglione M, et al. Long term results of 2 different ablation strategies in patients with paroxysmal and persistent atrial fibrillation. Circ Arrhythm Electrophysiol 2008; 1:269–275.
34. Hocini M, Jais P, Sanders P, et al. Techniques, evaluation, and consequences of linear block at the left atrial roof in paroxysmal atrial fibrillation: A prospective randomized study. Circulation 2005; 112:3688–3696.
35. Hsu LF, Jais P, Sanders P, et al. Catheter ablation for atrial fibrillation in congestive heart failure. N Engl J Med 2004; 351:2373–2383.

36. Jais P, Hocini M, Hsu LF, et al. Technique and results of linear ablation at the mitral isthmus. Circulation 2004; 110:2996–3002.

37. Cauchemez B, Haissaguerre M, Fischer B, Thomas O, Clementy J, Coumel P. Electrophysiological effects of catheter ablation of inferior vena cava-tricuspid annulus isthmus in common atrial flutter. Circulation 1996; 93:284–294.

38. Mesas C, Pappone C, Lang CCE, et al. Left atrial tachycardia after circumferential pulmonary vein ablation for atrial fibrillation: Electroanatomic characterization and treatment. J Am Coll Cardiol 2004; 44:1071–1079.

39. Chugh A, Oral H, Lemola K, et al. Prevalence, mechanisms, and clinical significance of macroreentrant atrial tachycardia during and following left atrial ablation for atrial fibrillation. Heart Rhythm 2005; 2:464–473.

40. Scherlag BJ, Yamanashi W, Patel U, Lazzara R, Jackman WM. Autonomically induced conversion of pulmonary vein focal firing into atrial fibrillation. J Am Coll Cardiol 2005; 45:1878–1886.

CHAPTER 5

Patient management pre-, during-, and postablation

David J. Wilber[1], Etienne Aliot[2], Edward B. Gerstenfeld[3], Chu-Pak Lau[4], Martin J. Schalij[5], Dipen Shah[6], Hans Kottkamp[7]

[1]Director of the Cardiology Department, Loyola University Medical Center, Chicago, IL, USA
[2]Cardio-vascular Diseases Department, CHU de Brabois, Vandoeuvre-lès-Nancy, France
[3]Cardiac Electrophysiology Department, University of California, San Francisco, CA, USA
[4]Cardiology Department, University of Hong Kong-Queen Mary Hospital, Hong Kong
[5]Cardiology Department, Leiden Hospital, Leiden, The Netherlands
[6]Cardiology Cantonal Hospital of Geneva, Geneva, Switzerland
[7]Herz-Zentrum, Hirslanden Clinic, Zürich, Switzerland

Preablation management

Anticoagulation
Effective anticoagulation therapy is often necessary before an ablation procedure for AF. The modalities and duration of preablation anticoagulation therapy are reported in detail in Chapter 6.

Other drugs
Drug treatment for nonarrhythmic indications is generally continued. There is no consensus with regard to discontinuing AADs, although to avoid confounding ablation effects with AAD effects, all AADs with the possible exception of amiodarone should be discontinued at least four half-lives in advance. However, if symptomatic arrhythmias demand, effective AADs may be continued.

Transesophageal echocardiogram
A preablation TEE is used to rule out the presence of a LA thrombus, and should be considered a supplementary and backup strategy to continuous effective anticoagulation leading up to the ablation procedure. It should be

Atrial Fibrillation Ablation, 2011 Update: The State of the Art based on the VeniceChart International Consensus Document, First Edition. Edited by Andrea Natale and Antonio Raviele.
© 2011 John Wiley & Sons, Ltd. Published 2011 by John Wiley & Sons, Ltd.

performed shortly before the ablation procedure and without an intervening window in effective anticoagulation. In many electrophysiological laboratories, TEE is performed only in patients presenting with AF and without Coumadin.

Other imaging studies
Imaging to define the cardiac substrate could include establishing the presence and extent of coronary artery disease (if present) and left ventricular size and function. A transthoracic echocardiogram before the procedure is useful and allows measurement of chamber size and ejection fraction.

Left atrial size is an important determinant of rhythm outcome after ablation and may influence the selection of ablation strategies. The most widely used measure, single-plane dimension from the parasternal long-axis view, correlates modestly with LA volumes. Estimation of LA volume from multiple 2D imaging planes or by volumetric analysis of MR or CT images may be preferable and more accurate.

Evaluation of left atrial emptying and systolic function (ejection fraction) is not part of most standard imaging routines but may have an important role in evaluating the long-term impact of ablation on left atrial function.

An MR or contrast-enhanced spiral CT scan is obtained as a baseline both for comparison and for formulation of an ablation strategy with variable PV anatomy [1]. In some laboratories, the ablation is performed with MR or CT image integration. In such situations, both the underlying rhythm and ventricular rate at the time of acquisition are important in order to make effective use of the 3D images [2]. Preliminary data indicate that preprocedure delayed enhancement MR may be useful in predicting procedural outcome [3].

Informed consent and preablation fasting

As for any ablation, an informed consent and appropriate preparation including at least 6 hours of fasting leading up to the procedure are necessary.

Management during ablation

Sedation/anesthesia
Conscious sedation using midazolam combined with analgesia using fentanyl is used in ablation procedures of less complex arrhythmias (e.g., AVN reentrant tachycardia) and can also be applied during AF ablation. However, conscious sedation is often inadequate during AF ablation due to long procedure times, pain during RF energy applications, and the need to limit patient motion during the procedure. Therefore, general anesthesia is widely used during AF ablation. General anesthesia may reduce the prevalence of PV reconnection during repeat ablation when compared with conscious sedation [4]. Alternatively, deep sedation during continuous infusion of propofol has evolved as a third sedation alternative. This strategy can achieve painless deep

sedation without the need for intubation and general anesthesia, and can be guided by the electrophysiologist [5].

Anticoagulation

The intensity of anticoagulation during the AF ablation is of critical importance and is described in Chapter 6.

Antiarrhythmic drugs/electrical cardioversion

Many investigators choose to perform the AF ablation procedure off AADs. The procedure can be performed during either sinus rhythm or AF. In selected cases, AADs may be administered intravenously when sinus rhythm is desired. Alternatively, electrical cardioversion can be applied when sinus rhythm is the preferred rhythm during specific parts of the procedure, e.g., verification of conduction block across linear ablation lines and confirmation of PV isolation.

Postprocedural management

The immediate postprocedural management consists of continuing and maintaining anticoagulation, maintaining hemostasis at puncture sites, and supportive treatment. Vagal episodes remedied by fluid infusion and/or atropine are not uncommon; however, pericardial tamponade must be excluded in patients with postprocedural hypotension. Pericarditic discomfort may occur during the first 3–5 days, sometimes accompanied by a mild and self-limited febrile syndrome. Aspirin is usually sufficient treatment although, uncommonly, continuing symptoms and a nonresolving pericardial effusion may require the administration of systemic steroids. The later occurrence (6–10 days postablation) of a febrile state with or without neurological symptoms should prompt suspicion of an atrioesophageal fistula and lead to a contrast-enhanced spiral CT to exclude the diagnosis.

Many centers now perform AF ablation while continuing therapeutic anticoagulation with warfarin [6]. In this case, oral warfarin anticoagulation can simply be continued after ablation. If warfarin is held for several days prior to ablation, bridging with intravenous unfractionated heparin or LMWH is typically performed until a therapeutic INR is achieved. A new alternative agent used for anticoagulation in AF is the direct thrombin inhibitor dabigatran [7]. There is no data yet available supporting the use of dabigatran during/after AF ablation. Because there is no agent available to reverse the anticoagulant effects of dabigatran, it is typically held 1–2 days prior to ablation and can be resumed orally on the evening or morning after ablation.

Rhythm outcome

Estimating the burden of AF, both symptomatic and asymptomatic, is the key to determining the outcome of the procedure. The ideal outcome would be a

Table 5.1 Incidence of asymptomatic AF in postablation patients.

Authors	Total number of patients	Number of patients with asymptomatic AF	Detection method
Oral et al. [8]	53	1 (2%)	TTEM
Hindricks et al. [9]	108	20 (18%)	7-d HM
Senatore et al. [10]	72	8 (11%)	TTEM
Neumann et al. [11]	80	11 (14%)	ELR
Vasamreddy et al. [12]	10	2 (20%)	MCOT
Klemm et al. [13]	80	7 (9%)	TTEM
Verma et al. [14]	86	2 (2%)	PM/ICD
Steven et al. [15]	37	0 (0%)	PM/ICD

Note: Only the incidence of asymptomatic episodes is reported.

zero residual burden with no AFL or atrial tachycardia. The absence of symptoms may not correspond to the stable restoration of sinus rhythm potentially due to ablation-induced denervation or because of the absence of symptoms at baseline. The accuracy of estimating AF burden depends chiefly upon the duration of ECG recording (Table 5.1) [8–15]. Many laboratories use a clinical definition of successful ablation to mean the absence of symptomatic tachycardia, as well as the absence of documented AF during periodic follow-up visits as well as on periodic 24–48-hour Holter recordings, typically at 1, 3, and 6 months after the ablation. An event recorder may be used to evaluate symptoms not elucidated by the above tests. However, extending the duration of Holter tracings to 7 days has been shown to enhance the sensitivity of detecting recurrent AF [16]. Another approach has been to monitor periodic, even daily, transtelephonic ECG recordings supplemented by ECG transmission during symptomatic episodes, although the correlation to AF burden may be difficult to determine [12]. Finally, more and more implanted devices have sufficient memory and accurate arrhythmia recognition software to provide probably the most accurate measurement of AF burden possible, but of course only in a limited patient population (Table 5.2) [17]. From a clinical standpoint, when success is defined as the restoration of stable sinus rhythm, this assumes the elimination of (sustained) atrial tachycardias as well, whether reentrant (flutters) or nonreentrant.

Table 5.2 Detection methods of asymptomatic AF.

Standard 12-lead ECG
24-h/7-day HM
In-hospital telemetry
Mobile continuous outpatient telemetry
Event recorder
Intermittent TTEM
External loop recorder
Implantable loop recorder
PM/ICD device memory

Owing to the difficulty of clinically measuring the AF burden, the temporal evolution of arrhythmias in ablated patients has not been clearly determined.

Although some groups have reablated patients as soon as they develop recurrent AF, others have advocated waiting for 1–3 months with or without adding AA treatment in the interim period. An early reablation may result (unnecessarily) in a higher incidence of local puncture site complications, a longer hospital stay, and the risks of an additional left-sided procedure. About 30–50% of patients with documented or symptomatic recurrences during the first 3 months after an AF ablation have no further AF or flutter even without additional ablation. However, early AF recurrences do portend a worse long-term outcome, and merit heightened awareness of later AF occurrences.

Antiarrhythmic therapy

It has been demonstrated in a prospective randomized trial that treatment with AADs during the first 6 weeks after AF ablation reduces the incidence of clinically significant atrial arrhythmias and need for cardioversion or hospitalization for arrhythmia management [18]. However, systematic antiarrhythmic drug therapy did not reduce late arrhythmia recurrence during longer term follow-up in the same population [19].

Alternatively, AADs are stopped four half-lives before ablation and not restarted unless symptomatic or sustained recurrences occur, particularly for patients not willing to undergo an additional procedure or at a high risk of arrhythmia recurrence. There are no guidelines for discontinuing AAD therapy. Depending upon the risk of recurrence and the accuracy of determining residual arrhythmias, trial of discontinuation may be offered after 3–6 arrhythmia free months. Other drugs such as angiotensin-converting enzyme inhibitors, angiotensin receptor blockers, statins, and polyunsaturated fatty acids may potentially prevent AF by a variety of mechanisms, including antifibrotic, anti-inflammatory, and antioxidant effects. However, the efficacy of these drugs in reducing postablation arrhythmia recurrences has yet to be demonstrated.

Late surveillance

Echocardiographic monitoring is useful to detect improvement in LVF and assess reductions in LA size after ablation [20,21]. In the light of the high rates of symptomatic PV stenosis/occlusion in the early days of ablation targeting the PVs, routine MR or CT imaging was advocated at 3–6 months following the ablation. However, improvements in intraprocedural imaging as well as strategic changes in placing ablation lesions more remote from the PV ostia has resulted in significant reductions in PV stenosis rates. Furthermore, about 80% of PV stenosis, including most single PV occlusions, are asymptomatic [22]. Consequently, routine imaging with MR or CT is often restricted to patients with suggestive symptoms. Finally, a significant risk of very late AF recurrence has been reported in several series [23,24]. Therefore, it is advisable to maintain periodic surveillance for arrhythmia recurrence at 6- or 12-month intervals, even in patients who are free of arrhythmias during the initial year following ablation.

References

1. Jongbloed MR, Bax JJ, Lamb HJ, et al. Multislice computed tomography versus intracardiac echocardiography to evaluate the pulmonary veins before radiofrequency catheter ablation of atrial fibrillation: A head-to-head comparison. J Am Coll Cardiol 2005; 45:343–350.
2. Dong J, Calkins H, Solomon SB, et al. Integrated electroanatomical mapping with three dimensional computed tomographic images for real-time guided ablations. Circulation 2006; 113:186–194.
3. Oakes RS, Badger TJ, Kholmovski EG, et al. Detection and quantification of left atrial structural remodeling with delayed-enhancement magnetic resonance imaging in patients with atrial fibrillation. Circulation 2009; 119:1758–1767.
4. Di Biase L, Conti S, Mohanty P, et al. General anesthesia reduces the prevalence of pulmonary vein reconnection during repeat ablation when compared with conscious sedation: Results from a randomized study. Heart Rhythm 2011; 8:368–372.
5. Kottkamp H, Hindricks G, Eitel C, et al. Deep sedation for catheter ablation of atrial fibrillation: A prospective study in 650 consecutive patients. J Cardiovasc Electrophysiol 2011 June 21. [Epub ahead of print]
6. Wazni OM, Beheiry S, Fahmy T, et al. Atrial fibrillation ablation in patients with therapeutic international normalized ratio: Comparison of strategies of anticoagulation management in the periprocedural period. Circulation 2007; 116:2531–2534.
7. Connolly SJ, Ezekowitz MD, Yusuf S, et al. Dagibatran versus warfarin in patients with atrial fibrillation. N Engl J Med 2009; 361: 1139–1151.
8. Oral H, Veerareddy S, Good E, et al. Prevalence of asymptomatic recurrences of atrial fibrillation after successful radiofrequency catheter ablation. J Cardiovasc Electrophysiol 2004; 15:920–924.
9. Hindricks G, Piorkowski C, Tanner H, et al. Perception of atrial fibrillation before and after radiofrequency catheter ablation: Relevance of asymptomatic arrhythmia recurrence. Circulation 2005; 112:307–313.
10. Senatore G, Stabile G, Bertaqglia E, et al. Role of transtelephonic electrocardiographic monitoring in detecting short-term arrhythmia recurrences after radiofrequency ablation in patients with atrial fibrillation. J Am Coll Cardiol 2005; 45:873–876.
11. Neumann T, Erdogan A, Dill T, et al. Asymptomatic recurrences of atrial fibrillation after pulmonary vein isolation. Europace 2006; 8:495–498.
12. Vasamreddy CR, Dalal D, Dong J, et al. Symptomatic and asymptomatic atrial fibrillation in patients undergoing radiofrequency catheter ablation. J Cardiovasc Electrophysiol 2006; 17:134–139.
13. Klemm HU, Ventura R, Rostock T, et al. Correlation of symptoms to ECG diagnosis following atrial fibrillation ablation. J Cardiovasc Electrophysiol 2006; 17:146–150.
14. Verma A, Minor S, Kilicaslan F, et al. Incidence of atrial arrhythmias detected by permanent pacemakers (PPM) post-pulmonary vein antrum isolation (PVAI) for atrial fibrillation (AF): Correlation with symptomatic recurrence. J Cardiovasc Electrophysiol 2007; 18:601–606.

15. Steven D, Rostock T, Lutomsky B, et al. What is the real atrial fibrillation burden after catheter ablation of atrial fibrillation? A prospective rhythm analysis in pacemaker patients with continuous atrial monitoring. Eur Heart J 2008; 29:1037–1042.
16. Kottkamp H, Tanner H, Kobza R, et al. Time course and quantitative analysis of atrial fibrillation episode number and duration after circular plus linear left atrial lesions: Trigger elimination or substrate modification; early or delayed cure? J Am Coll Cardiol 2004; 44:869–877.
17. Capucci A, Santini M, Padeletti, et al. for the Italian AT 500 Registry Investigators. Monitored atrial fibrillation duration predicts arterial embolic events in patients suffering from bradycardia and atrial fibrillation implanted with antitachycardia pacemakers. J Am Coll Cardiol 2005; 46:1913–1920.
18. Roux JF, Zado E, Callans DJ, et al. Antiarrhythmics After Ablation of Atrial Fibrillation (5A Study). Circulation 2009; 120:1036–1040.
19. Leong-Sit P, Roux JF, Zado E, et al. Antiarrhythmics After Ablation of Atrial Fibrillation (5A Study): Six-Month Follow-Up Study. Circ Arrhythm Electrophysiol 2011; 4:11–14.
20. Verma A, Kilicaslan F, Adams JR, et al. Extensive ablation during pulmonary vein antrum isolation has no adverse impact of left atrial function: An echocardiography and cine computed tomography analysis. J Cardiovasc Electrophysiol 2006; 17:741–746.
21. Reant P, Lafitte S, Jais P, et al. Reverse remodelling of the left cardiac chambers after catheter ablation after 1 year in a series of patients with isolated atrial fibrillation. Circulation 2005; 112:2896–2903.
22. Di Biase L, Fahmy TS, Wazni OM, et al. Pulmonary vein total occlusion following catheter ablation for atrial fibrillation: Clinical implications after long-term follow-up. J Am Coll Cardiol 2006; 48:2493–2499.
23. Bertaglia E, Tondo C, De Simone A, et al. Does catheter ablation cure atrial fibrillation? Single-procedure outcome of drug-refractory atrial fibrillation ablation: A 6-year multicentre experience. Europace 2010; 12:181–187.
24. Wokhlu A, Hodge DO, Monahan KH, et al. Long-term outcome of atrial fibrillation ablation: Impact and predictors of very late recurrence. J Cardiovasc Electrophysiol 2010; 21:1071–1078.

Periprocedural and long-term anticoagulation

Stuart J. Connolly[1], David Callans[2], Mélèze Hocini[3], Gregory Y.H. Lip[4], Gregory F. Michaud[5], Albert L. Waldo[6], Sakis Themistoclakis[7]

[1]Cardiology Department, McMaster University, Hamilton, ON, Canada
[2]Cardiovascular Disease Department, Hospital of the University of Pennsylvania, Philadelphia, PA, USA
[3]Cardiology Department, Hôpital Haut-Lévêque, CHU de Bordeaux, Bordeaux, France
[4]University Department of Medicine, City Hospital, Birmingham, UK
[5]Center for Advanced Management of Atrial Fibrillation, Brigham and Women's Hospital, Boston, MA, USA
[6]Harrington-McLaughlin Heart & Vascular Institute, Division of Cardiovascular Medicine, University Hospitals Case Medical Center, Cleveland, OH, USA
[7]Cardiovascular Department, Dell'Angelo Hospital, Mestre, Italy

Introduction

Stroke is by far the most serious adverse consequence of AF, and concern about stroke prevention pervades all decision-making related to management of AF, including ablation. Although the primary motivation for PVI procedures is to reduce symptoms, nonetheless, stroke prevention needs to be considered before, during, and after ablation procedures for AF. This chapter considers these issues. Pre- and periprocedural anticoagulation is widely practiced. There are no controlled trials examining how best to reduce embolic and thrombotic complications, nor how to minimize the risk of hemorrhage. Such studies are needed. In the interim, it is prudent to follow current practice related to periprocedural anticoagulation. A more controversial issue is related to long-term anticoagulation following an apparently successful ablation procedure. In low-risk patients, long-term anticoagulation usually is not indicated. In moderate and especially higher risk patients, the question of long-term anticoagulation is difficult. The greatest difficulty is related to the lack of reliable information, particularly from randomized controlled trials. In the absence of reliable data supporting discontinuation of anticoagulation

Atrial Fibrillation Ablation, 2011 Update: The State of the Art based on the VeniceChart International Consensus Document, First Edition. Edited by Andrea Natale and Antonio Raviele.
© 2011 John Wiley & Sons, Ltd. Published 2011 by John Wiley & Sons, Ltd.

in high-risk patients, it is prudent to continue long-term anticoagulation, despite some follow-up studies suggesting a low risk of stroke, as retrospective nonrandomized studies are inherently unreliable.

In the last year, there have been important advances in anticoagulant therapy for the prevention of stroke in AF. Information from large randomized trials is now becoming rapidly available indicating that new anticoagulants will be effective against stroke in AF. In particular, dabigatran has been shown to be more effective than warfarin with a lower risk of bleeding and with a greater ease of use. The availability of dabigatran in most countries makes it more acceptable to continue long-term anticoagulation after apparently successful ablation in patients with moderate to high risk for stroke.

None of the recommendations in this chapter are based on the results of randomized controlled trials and, therefore, all must be taken as somewhat provisional. This points to the great need for rigorously designed and carefully executed studies of anticoagulation before, during and especially after, PV ablation for AF.

Preablation anticoagulation and TEE

Because AF ablation involves not only cardioversion in many patients and the introduction of foreign bodies into the left heart but also the possibility of a lapse in anticoagulation during sheath removal, the importance of preprocedural anticoagulation is well accepted. However, there are many potential strategies and very little data to guide best practices.

Anticoagulation strategies prior to ablation procedures in high-risk patients reflect guidelines for the care of patients with AF in general. Patients with CHADS$_2$ scores of 2 or higher should be anticoagulated in any case to an INR of 2–3 for at least 3 weeks prior to ablation; if warfarin is stopped prior to the procedure, enoxaparin or heparin may be used for "bridging." There is little consensus regarding the need for anticoagulation in low-risk patients. Recent observational studies suggest that a strategy of performing ablation with a therapeutic INR may reduce the risk of ablation-related thromboembolism [1,2]. This strategy has the theoretical advantage of eliminating the lapse in anticoagulation during sheath removal, and has been shown to be associated with a low rate of bleeding complications and of periprocedural stroke. The impact of new oral anticoagulants has not been studied in this application.

Many centers routinely perform TEE prior to ablation to exclude the presence of thrombus in high-risk patients, particularly in those with persistent AF. Other strategies to assess the presence of thrombus, such as computed tomographic angiography, or intraprocedural ICE, may be reasonable but have not been rigorously compared to TEE, which is the current gold standard. There is little consensus in low-risk patients, or those with paroxysmal AF. A recent paper suggested that the incidence of intracardiac thrombus was low in ablation candidates (0.6%), but increased with increasing CHADS$_2$ score, history of heart failure, and LVEF <35% [3].

Recommendations (based on expert opinion and small observational studies):

1 In patients at moderate to high risk of stroke, anticoagulation with a vitamin K antagonist (INR 2–3, target 2.5) or a new anticoagulant is recommended for 3 weeks prior to ablation. For patients at low risk of stroke, the need for this is unknown.

2 TEE or other methods to exclude intracardiac thrombus prior to ablation is recommended in patients with persistent AF or other high-risk characteristics.

Anticoagulation during the ablation procedure

In the updated worldwide survey of catheter ablation for AF, a 0.94% incidence of stroke or TIA was reported [4]; however, an 11–14% incidence of silent cerebral emboli were observed following catheter ablation in two recently published studies [5,6]. Major bleeding complications such as tamponade, hemothorax, and groin complications such as pseudoaneurysm or AV fistula totaled 2.3%. Femoral hematomas are more common, up to 8% [7], and may prolong hospitalization or produce a short period of disability. Achieving the lowest possible thromboembolic complication rate while maintaining an acceptably low bleeding complication rate is the goal of intraprocedural anticoagulation. Thrombus can form within sheaths or on guidewires and catheters, as observed by ICE (Figure 6.1), particularly in patients with persistent AF, dilated atria, and spontaneous echo contrast [8]. To prevent thrombus formation within the sheaths, it is common sense to flush them intermittently or use continuous irrigation, which may be more reliable. Since the capacity of

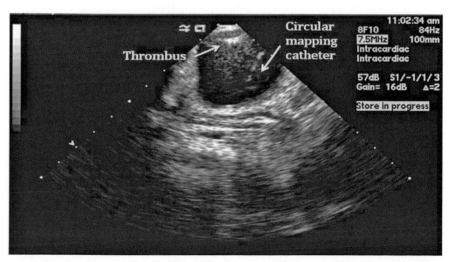

Figure 6.1 Image from an intracardiac echocardiogram showing a CMC in the LA with a mobile thrombus attached.

the inner lumen for blood is larger without a catheter in place, it may be beneficial to leave catheters in sheaths while in the LA. Endocardial RFCA may disrupt endothelial integrity and expose a nidus of interstitial tissue, which may promote thrombus formation. Char may form on the electrodes of the ablation catheter if temperatures exceed 100°C at the electrode–tissue interface, which may increase the risk of thrombus formation. A sudden impedance rise during RF energy delivery may indicate the development of char and should prompt withdrawal and inspection of the catheter tip. A catheter tip with open irrigation appears to reduce the risk of char and thrombus formation by cooling the electrode–tissue interface [9].

Unfractionated heparin, delivered by weight/time-based nomograms and/or monitored by frequent measurement of ACT, is typically given during the ablation procedure, even in the presence of a therapeutic INR (thrombus may form in the RA with similar frequency as it does in patients with an INR < 2.0) [10]. Exchanging short vascular access sheaths for transseptal sheaths should be preceded by careful flushing and heparin delivery should be considered at this point rather than after TSP, particularly in patients with a higher risk of thromboembolism. The target intensity of anticoagulation is not standardized among experienced investigators, and may vary according to several factors, for example, patient age, type of ablation procedure, catheter used, and energy source. Observational studies have shown using ICE that the incidence of visualized thrombus markedly decreased with an increase in target ACT from 250–300 to >300 seconds [8,11]. Many experienced operators instruct their patients to maintain a therapeutic INR, as it may be easier to achieve and maintain target ACT values and may reduce the risk of stroke. The risk of major bleeding complications does not appear to increase using this strategy [7,12]. Additionally, management of cardiac tamponade appears to be equally safe in patients with a therapeutic INR, but reversal agents such as fresh frozen plasma or factor IX should be readily available during the procedure if a therapeutic INR is to be maintained [13].

Recommendations (based on expert opinion and small observational studies):

1 Heparin administration should be initiated at the time of the exchange of short vascular sheaths for transseptal sheaths, and no later than immediately after TSP is safely accomplished.

2 Heparin should be administered as an initial bolus dose of 100–140 IU/kg followed by an infusion of 15–18 IU/(kg h) and/or by additional boluses. For patients with an INR range of 2.0–3.5, the initial bolus dose should be reduced to 80 IU/kg.

3 The ACT target should be 350–400 seconds based on limited data. The ACT target does not differ in patients with and without a therapeutic INR.

4 Heparin infusion is discontinued in all patients after removal of catheters from the LA. Protamine infusion may be administered (dose 30–50 mg) or ACT allowed to decrease below 250 seconds prior to sheath removal to minimize the potential for femoral hematoma formation.

Postablation anticoagulation

No universally accepted recommendations exist for anticoagulation therapy after successful ablation of AF. Due to the high risk of thromboembolism in the early postprocedural period [14], in the many centers, warfarin therapy, if interrupted before the procedure, is started in all patients either the same evening of the ablation procedure or the next morning. In the initial period, LMWH (e.g., enoxaparin at a dosage of 0.5–1.0 mg/kg twice a day) is often given as bridging therapy by starting 3–4 hours after the ablation [15,16]. Less frequently, heparin is administered intravenously until the day after the procedure, starting about 3 hours after sheath removal at a rate of 1000 IU/h [14,17]. Thereafter, LMWH is administrated until the INR is ≥ 2. Warfarin is usually continued for at least 3 months. Bunch et al. recently reported that selected low-risk patients (CHADS$_2$ score ≤ 1), who undergo left atrial ablation with an aggressive anticoagulation strategy with heparin and use of an open irrigated tip catheter, can safely be discharged following their procedure on aspirin alone [18]. However, the results of this observational single center study, conducted in a small population, need to be confirmed in larger prospective randomized trial before to be considered in the clinical practice

The anticoagulation strategy after the initial 3 months is controversial. There have been several reports indicating that a low rate of stroke may occur in patients with successful ablation who do not receive anticoagulation. However, none of these provide randomized data.

Oral et al. reported that none of the 383 patients who had suspended warfarin in the absence of arrhythmic recurrences suffered any TE during a 24-month follow-up, while 2 of the 357 patients who remained on OAC after ablation had a TEs (0.56%) [14]. Moreover, two cerebral hemorrhages (0.56%) occurred among the patients on OAC. It should, however, be pointed out that in this study two important categories of high-risk patients (over 65 years of age or with a preablation history of stroke) were underrepresented (only 49 and 10 patients, respectively) and that these patients were often maintained on OAC. In a study of long-term outcomes after AF substrate ablation guided by CFAEs, Nademanee et al. compared the incidence of TEs and hemorrhages between 434 patients without arrhythmic recurrences who discontinued warfarin and 118 patients requiring OAC following unsuccessful ablation [19]. These patients were selected from a cohort of patients who were at least 65 years old or had 1 or more risk factors for stroke, including hypertension, diabetes, SHD, prior history of stroke/TIA, CHF, or LVEF $\leq 40\%$. In their population, the annual stroke rate was significantly lower in successfully treated patients who discontinued warfarin than in patients with AF recurrences who remained on OAC therapy (0.4% vs. 2%). Corrado et al. in a study of 138 septuagenarians successfully treated with AF ablation and followed up for 16 ± 12 months after OAC discontinuation, observed that none suffered thromboembolism [20]. Finally, Themistoclakis et al. in a recent, larger, multicenter study enrolled 3355 patients, of whom 2692 discontinued OAC 3–6 months after successful ablation off AADs in absence of severe left atrial dysfunction or severe PV stenosis [21]. CHADS$_2$ scores of 1 and $\geq$2 were recorded in 723 and 347 patients who discontinued warfarin, respectively. In this study, after about 2 years of follow-up, the percentage of TEs in patients who suspended warfarin following successful AF ablation was not significantly different from that observed in patients who continued warfarin after the procedure (0.07% vs. 0.45%, respectively; $p = .06$). Moreover, the incidence of major hemorrhages was significantly lower among patients who suspended warfarin than among those who continued (0.04% vs. 2% respectively; $p < .0001$).

These studies have the following limitations: (1) they are observational, retrospective, and nonrandomized, and (2) most enrolled few patients at high thromboembolic risk. In addition, there may be publication bias as these reports have been retrospective.

The reasons for continuing anticoagulation after ablation mainly concern the risk of long-term recurrence [22–27] and in particular, the risk of asymptomatic recurrences [28]. Furthermore, it is generally accepted that there is a continuing risk of stroke in patients receiving AAD therapy even if it appears that therapy has eliminated AF recurrences. Therefore, it would appear to be prudent at this point to recommend that long-term anticoagulation be continued in patients even after apparently successful ablation. The use of anticoagulation requires an assessment of stroke risk and bleeding risk as well as patient values. Aspirin is generally considered a poor substitute for OAC. New anticoagulants such as dabigatran, which is easier to use than warfarin, more effective, and associated with fewer life-threatening bleeds, make the decision to continue an anticoagulant after apparently successful ablation more attractive.

Recommendations (based on expert opinion and small observational studies):

1 OAC should be started after ablation and continued for at least 3 months in all patients.

2 OAC should be continued indefinitely in most patients who are at moderate or high risk of stroke (based on a risk stratification system such as CHADS$_2$ or CHA$_2$DS$_2$-VASc). This recommendation is based on a known risk of AF recurrence, and a lack of randomized, prospectively obtained trial data indicating the safety of anticoagulation discontinuation.

3 New anticoagulants, such as dabigatran, can be used instead of vitamin K antagonists and may be preferred due to improved benefit-risk profiles.

References

1. Hussein AA, Martin DO, Saliba W, et al. Radiofrequency ablation of atrial fibrillation under therapeutic international normalized ratio: A safe and efficacious periprocedural anticoagulation strategy. Heart Rhythm 2009; 6:1425–1429.
2. Di Biase L, Burkhardt JD, Mohanty P, et al. Periprocedural stroke and management of major bleeding complications in patients undergoing catheter ablation of atrial

fibrillation: The impact of periprocedural therapeutic international normalized ratio. Circulation 2010; 121:2550–2556.

3. Puwanant S, Varr BC, Shrestha K, et al. Role of the CHADS2 score in the evaluation of thromboembolic risk in patients with atrial fibrillation undergoing transesophageal echocardiography before pulmonary vein isolation. J Am Coll Cardiol 2009; 54:2032–2039.

4. Cappato R, Calkins H, Chen SA, et al. Updated worldwide survey on the methods, efficacy, and safety of catheter ablation for human atrial fibrillation. Circ Arrhythm Electrophysiol 2010; 3:32–38.

5. Schrickel JW, Lickfett L, Lewalter T, et al. Incidence and predictors of silent cerebral embolism during pulmonary vein catheter ablation for atrial fibrillation. Europace 2010; 12:52–57.

6. Gaita F, Caponi D, Pianelli M, et al. Radiofrequency catheter ablation of atrial fibrillation: A cause of silent thromboembolism? Magnetic resonance imaging assessment of cerebral thromboembolism in patients undergoing ablation of atrial fibrillation. Circulation 2010; 122:1667–1673.

7. Gautam S, John RJ, Stevenson WG, et al. Effect of therapeutic INR on activated clotting times, heparin dosage and bleeding risk during ablation of atrial fibrillation. J Cardiovasc Electrophysiol 2011; 22:248–254.

8. Ren JF, Marchlinski FE, Callans DJ, et al. Increased intensity of anticoagulation may reduce risk of thrombus during atrial fibrillation ablation procedures in patients with spontaneous echo contrast. J Cardiovasc Electrophysiol 2005; 16:474–477.

9. Yokoyama K, Nakagawa H, Wittkampf F. Comparison of electrode cooling between internal and open irrigation in radiofrequency ablation lesion depth and incidence of thrombus and steam pop. Circulation 2006; 113:11–19.

10. Di Biase L, Mohanty P, Sanchez J. Prevalence of right atrial thrombus on the transseptal sheaths detected by intracardiac echocardiography during catheter ablation for atrial fibrillation while on therapeutic Coumadin. AHA 2010, Vol. 122, Abstract 17354.

11. Wazni OM, Rossillo A, Marrouche NF, et al. Embolic events and char formation during pulmonary vein isolation in patients with atrial fibrillation: Impact of different anticoagulation regimens and importance of intracardiac echo imaging. J Cardiovasc Electrophysiol 2005; 16:576–581.

12. Di Biase L, Burkhardt JD, Mohanty P, et al. Risk of stroke in patients with and without a therapeutic INR. Circulation 2010; 121:2550–2556.

13. Latchamsetty R, Gautam S, Bhakta D, et al. Management and outcomes of cardiac tamponade during atrial fibrillation ablation in the presence of therapeutic anticoagulation with warfarin. Heart Rhythm 2011; 8:805–808.

14. Oral H, Chugh A, Ozaydin M, et al. Risk of thromboembolic events after percutaneous left atrial radiofrequency ablation of atrial fibrillation. Circulation 2006; 114:759–765.

15. Verma A, Marrouche NF, Natale A. Pulmonary vein antrum isolation: Intracardiac echocardiography-guided technique. J Cardiovasc Electrophysiol 2004; 15:1335–1340.

16. Haïssaguerre M, Hocini M, Sanders P, et al. Catheter ablation of long-lasting persistent atrial fibrillation: Clinical outcome and mechanisms of subsequent arrhythmias. J Cardiovasc Electrophysiol 2005; 16:1138—1147.

17. Pappone C, Santinelli V. How to perform encircling ablation of the left atrium. Heart Rhythm 2006; 3:1105–1109.

18. Bunch TJ, Crandall BG, Weiss JP, et al. Warfarin is not needed in low-risk patients following atrial fibrillation ablation procedures. J Cardiovasc Electrophysiol 2009; 20:988–993.

19. Nademanee K, Schwab MC, Kosar EM, et al. Clinical outcomes of catheter substrate ablation for high-risk patients with atrial fibrillation. J Am Coll Cardiol 2008; 51:843–849.

20. Corrado A, Patel D, Riedlbauchova L, et al. Efficacy, safety, and outcome of atrial fibrillation ablation in septuagenarians. J Cardiovasc Electrophysiol 2008; 19:807–811.

21. Themistoclakis S, Corrado A, Marchlinski FE, et al. The risk of thromboembolism and need for oral anticoagulation after successful atrial fibrillation ablation. J Am Coll Cardiol 2010; 55.735–743.

22. Natale A, Raviele A, Arentz T, et al. Venice chart international consensus document on atrial fibrillation ablation. J Cardiovasc Electrophysiol 2007; 18:560–580.

23. Katritsis D, Wood MA, Giazitzoglou E, Shepard RK, Kourlaba G, Ellenbogen KA. Long-term follow-up after radiofrequency catheter ablation for atrial fibrillation. Europace 2008; 10:419–424.

24. Bertaglia E, Tondo C, De Simone A, et al. Does catheter ablation cure atrial fibrillation? Single-procedure outcome of drug-refractory atrial fibrillation ablation: A 6-year multicentre experience. Europace 2010; 12:181–187.

25. Wokhlu A, Hodge DO, Monahan KH, et al. Long-term outcome of atrial fibrillation ablation: Impact and predictors of very late recurrence J Cardiovasc Electrophysiol 2010; 21:1071–1078.

26. Ouyang F, Tilz R, Chun J, Schmidt B, et al. Long-term results of catheter ablation in paroxysmal atrial fibrillation: Lessons from a 5-year follow-up. Circulation 2010; 122:2368–2377.

27. Bhargava M, Di Biase L, Mohanty P, et al. Impact of type of atrial fibrillation and repeat catheter ablation on long-term freedom from atrial fibrillation: Results from a multicenter study. Heart Rhythm 2009; 6:1403–1412.

28. Kuck KH, Shah D, Camm AJ, et al. Patient management pre- and postablation In: Natale A, Raviele A, eds. *Atrial Fibrillation Ablation*. Malden, MA: Blackwell Futura; 2007, pp. 34–40.

CHAPTER 7

Periprocedural and late complications

Francis E. Marchlinski[1], Thomas Arentz[2], Rodney P. Horton[3], Hakan Oral[4], Antonio Rossillo[5], Eduardo Saad[6], Mauricio Scanavacca[7], Riccardo Cappato[8]

[1]Cardiovascular Division, Hospital of the University of Pennsylvania, Philadelphia, PA, USA
[2]Rhythmology Department, Herz-Zentrum, Bad Krozingen, Germany
[3]Texas Cardiac Arrhythmia Institute, St. David's Medical Center, Austin, TX, USA
[4]Cardiovascular Medicine Department, University of Michigan, Ann Arbor, MI, USA
[5]Cardiovascular Department, Dell'Angelo Hospital, Venice-Mestre, Italy
[6]Center for Atrial Fibrillation, Pro-Cardiaco Hospital, Rio de Janeiro, Brazil
[7]Heart Institute, University of Sao Paulo Medical School, Sao Paulo, Brazil
[8]Electrophysiology Department, Policlinico S. Donato, San Donato Milanese, Italy

Recognition of common and unique complications related to AF ablation, their incidence, etiology, and techniques for prevention can minimize risk and optimize the outcome of the ablation procedure. A reasonable and current estimate of risk in the general electrophysiology community has been suggested from the updated worldwide survey based on experience with over 16,000 patients undergoing catheter ablation for AF and from detailed, large single-center experiences [1–4] (Table 7.1). This section will provide and updated review of each of the major/unique complications related to the AF ablation procedure (Table 7.2).

Cardiac tamponade

Pericardial effusion/tamponade is a potential complication of all catheter-based cardiac procedures [5,6]. As catheter ablation of AF was not routinely performed when early catheter ablation registries were published, the question arises whether left atrial ablation of AF carries an inherent higher risk of pericardial effusion and cardiac tamponade [5,6]. Published worldwide survey investigating methods, efficacy and safety of catheter ablation of AF [7] represents the widest available source of information concerning complications of AF catheter ablation. Among 8754 patients who underwent catheter

Atrial Fibrillation Ablation, 2011 Update: The State of the Art based on the VeniceChart International Consensus Document, First Edition. Edited by Andrea Natale and Antonio Raviele.
© 2011 John Wiley & Sons, Ltd. Published 2011 by John Wiley & Sons, Ltd.

Table 7.1 Worldwide survey of complications reported in catheter ablation studies

Type of Complication	No. of Patients	Rate, %
Death	25	0.15
Tamponade	213	1.31
Pneumothorax	15	0.09
Hemothorax	4	0.02
Sepsis, abscesses, or endocarditis	2	0.01
Permanent diaphragmatic paralysis	28	0.17
Total femoral pseudoaneurysm	152	0.93
Total artero-venous fistulae	88	0.54
Valve damage/requiring surgery	11/7	0.07
Atrium-esophageal fistulae	6	0.04
Stroke	37	0.23
Transient ischemic attack	115	0.71
PV stenoses requiring intervention	48	0.29
Total	741	4.54

Source: Reproduced from Cappato R, Calkins H, Chen SA, et al. Updated worldwide survey on the methods, efficacy, and safety of catheter ablation for human AF. Circ Arrhythm Electrphysiol 2010; 3:32–38.

ablation of AF between 1995 and 2002, periprocedural cardiac tamponade occurred in 107 patients (1.2%). Aside from chronic PV stenosis, cardiac tamponade was the most common procedure-related major complication in this original survey. A rate of 0.0–1.3% of cardiac tamponade has been reported in single center series of patients who underwent PV antral isolation [2,6–9]. A persistent risk of above 1% have been confirmed in a recent worldwide report update investigating clinical outcome in 16,309 patients undergoing 20,823 procedures performed in the years between 2003 and 2006 [7]. In this series, cardiac tamponade was reported in 1.31% of all procedures. Compared with the previous survey, this figure was observed despite a higher degree of procedure complexity and larger proportion of catheter ablation of persistent and long-standing persistent AF. A stable incidence of tamponade suggests a higher degree of safety associated with catheter ablation of AF in the recent years in doing procedures that in general have used more catheter manipulation and lesion formation.

Clinical manifestations of acute tamponade include hypotension, tachycardia, dyspnea, paradoxical pulse, jugular venous distension, and shock. Constant vigilance with access to echocardiographic imaging and experience in gaining pericardial access for prompt drainage may be lifesaving. If not correctly recognized and promptly treated, cardiac tamponade can lead to irreversible circulatory collapse and death. In a recent multicenter series, cardiac tamponade was found to be the most common cause of periprocedural death, with 22% of all reported fatalities being observed as a consequence of this complication [10]. Occasionally, open-heart surgery,

Table 7.2 Complications of AF ablation.

Complication	Incidence	Cause	Clinical presentation	Diagnostic tools	Prevention	Therapy
Cardiac tamponade	0.0–2.9%	TSP Linear lesions High RF power	Chest pain Tachycardia Dyspnea Abrupt Hypotension/shock	TTE	ICE-guided procedure Power limitation Avoidance of RF delivery in CS	Pericardiocentesis Surgical drainage
TEs	0.20–0.94%	Use of number of sheaths/catheters in the arterial system Wide disruption of LA endocardial surface	Neurological deficits Acute ischemia of different organs depending on the site of thromboembolism	Head CT/MR imaging Different tools	Intermittent flush or continuous irrigations of the sheaths Intravenous heparin administration with an ACT targeted of 250–400 Use of open irrigated tip catheters	Different according to the organ site of the thromboembolism
PV stenosis	0.5–2%	RF delivery inside PVs	Cough Dyspnea Hemoptysis Recurrent/drug resistant pneumonia	Transesophageal echocardiography V/Q lung scan CT/MR imaging	Use of imaging techniques Impedance measurements Titration of energy delivery	Anticoagulation Angioplasty/ stenting Surgery
PN injury	0.1–0.5%	RF delivery at sites in close proximity to right/left PN (RSPV, SVC, etc.)	Dyspnea Cough Weakness Unilateral diaphragmatic paralysis	Fluoroscopy	Avoidance of energy application at sites of high-output pacing-induced diaphragmatic contraction	No therapy (spontaneous recovery)

(Continued)

Table 7.2 (*Continued*)

Complication	Incidence	Cause	Clinical presentation	Diagnostic tools	Prevention	Therapy
Atrioesophageal fistula	0.03–0.25%	RF delivery at posterior wall of LA	Fever Malaise Dysphagia Hematemesis/melena Neurological deficits Intermittent cardiac ischemia Septic shock	CT/MR imaging	Monitoring of esophageal location/temperature Avoidance of micro bubble formation Low-energy delivery for short duration	Surgical correction Stenting of the esophagus
Periesophageal vagal injury	1%	Injury of periesophageal vagal plexus	Abdominal bloating Discomfort Pain	Gastroscopy and upper gastrointestinal investigation	Esophageal temperature monitoring Power titration and limitation at posterior LA	Endoscopic intrapiloric botulinum toxic injection
Vascular complications (groin hematoma, pseudoaneurysm, AV fistula, retroperitoneal bleeding)	0–13%	Use of numerous venous catheters Routine use of femoral arterial line Intense use of anticoagulation	Local symptoms/ signs Anemia	Echography	Procedure performance on oral anticoagulation Use of ultrasound-guided access Use of micropuncture kits Avoidance of large sheaths Adequate vascular compression	Transfusion if necessary Echo-guided manual compression/ Thrombin injection Surgical intervention

Acute circumflex artery occlusion	0.002%	RF delivery in the distal part of CS	Chest pain ST-segment elevation	ECG coronary angiography	More posterior placement of mitral isthmus linear lesions Power limitation	Standard therapy of acute coronary artery occlusion
Air emboli	?[a]	Sheaths/catheters exchanges Aspiration/irrigation/ continuous infusion of sheaths	Symptoms/signs of acute myocardial ischemia Neurological manifestations	ECG/coronary angiography Head CT/MR imaging	Proper attention to the technique	Standard therapy of air emboli Hyperbaric oxygen
Catheter entrapment in the MV	0.01%	Inadvertent positioning of the CMC into the ventricle	No specific symptoms/signs	Echocardiography	Posterior TSP Clockwise catheter rotation when leaving transseptal sheath	Gentle catheter manipulation Advancement of sheath over the catheter into the ventricle Surgical extraction
Left AFL/ tachycardia	3–40%	Reconnection of previously isolated PVs Slow conduction induced by incomplete linear lesions	Palpitations	ECG	Complete PV isolation Avoidance of linear lesions Documentation of bidirectional block in case of linear lesions	AA drugs Redo ablation

[a] ? means "unknown/not reported."

including cardio-pulmonary by-pass may be required for the treatment of cardiac tamponade [11].

Tamponade risk related to TSP appears to be related to experience with the technique. Monitoring tools such as intracardiac or transesophageal echo with direct visualization of the TSP may help minimize risk related to experience. Direct echocardiographic imaging can identify unique anatomic variants such as septal aneurysms, hypertrophied atrial septum or thickened/fibrosed fossa ovalis that may increase technical difficulty [12]. Of note, a recent multicenter survey on transseptal catheterization spanning 12 years [13] reported a very low incidence of cardiac tamponade complicating LA catheterization performed for ablation of various arrhythmic substrates (5 cardiac tamponade in 5520 procedures; 0.1%). Therefore, it seems reasonable to assume that RF energy delivery and complicated catheter manipulation in the region of the LAA also contribute significantly to the risk of cardiac tamponade during catheter ablation of AF. In a series of 348 irrigated-tip AF ablations with complete PVs isolation including left atrial linear ablation in 254 and cavotricuspid isthmus ablation in 265, 10 patients (2.9%) suffered cardiac tamponade during the procedure [14]. All tamponade occurred during linear ablation attempting to create bidirectional conduction block in either the left or the RA. In 8 out of 10 patients cardiac tamponade was associated with "popping", consistent with tissue disruption. A comparative analysis between patients with and without tamponade revealed that RF power was significantly higher in patients who developed tamponade (53 ± 4 vs. 48 ± 7 W). The subsequent decision to limit power delivery to ≤42 W during linear ablation reduced the incidence of cardiac tamponade to 1% (4 cardiac tamponade among the subsequent 398 procedures). A further power limitation to ≤40 W resulted in no cardiac tamponade in the next 167 AF ablations.

Recently, cases of delayed cardiac tamponade (i.e., occurring after patient discharge from the electrophysiological laboratory or from hospital) have been reported, sometimes preceded by evidence of pericarditis [15]. Similar to what is observed with intraprocedural cardiac tamponade, pericardiocentesis represents the appropriate therapy for this complication. Data for a more systematic evaluation about the causes, treatment and outcome of delayed cardiac tamponade await results of a more detailed dedicated ongoing multicenter survey that focuses on this complication.

Although identification of the possible causes of cardiac tamponade is made difficult by its low occurrence, a repeat procedure with AF recurrence has been suggested to increase by a factor of 3 the risk of this and other complications [14]. Importantly, a recent study from a single high-volume center experience suggests that patients with cardiac tamponade during ablation procedure in the context of ongoing oral anticoagulants do not have a higher risk of ominous outcome as compared with patients in whom this therapy is discontinued before ablation [16].

Thus, although in some patients cardiac tamponade results from mechanical trauma from TSP or catheter manipulation careful titration of RF power delivery seems to reduce tissue boiling and endocardial rupture and further reduce risk. The role of catheter tip contact force sensing on risk assessment for tamponade with catheter manipulation and the use of stiffer steerable sheaths during energy delivery is being actively evaluated. The use of remote navigation systems is also being evaluated to determine the potential for risk reduction.

Thromboembolic events

The prevalence of TEs during or after AF ablation has been reported to vary between 0.20% and 0.94% in recent studies. [1,3,17,18]. The effects of AF ablation on the risk of TEs may be quite complex from a mechanistic perspective, these effects may be best examined by dividing the TEs into early and late postablation events.

Early Postablation thromboembolic events

Early postoperative TEs, i.e., those occurring during or within 30 days after an ablation procedure are usually related to procedural and/or technical factors. During AF ablation, a relatively long (often >3–4 hours) procedure is performed in the arterial system utilizing a number of sheaths, guidewires, and catheters. Furthermore, RF energy is widely applied to the endocardial surface to interfere with the excitability and conductivity of the underlying atrial tissue. TEs may occur due to a variety of mechanisms.

Thrombus may form within or over the catheters, guidewires or sheaths during the course of an ablation procedure. To prevent thrombus formation within the sheaths, it is important to flush the sheaths intermittently or to use continuous irrigation as previously described. It may also be helpful to not leave sheaths without a catheter inside in the LA. Appropriate anticoagulation should be rapidly achieved as soon as the TSP is made. Systemic anticoagulation just prior to the TSP (after confirming the needle position with ICE) has also been used to minimize the risk of thrombus formation. Left atrial thrombi can be detected by ICE and appear to be more likely to form on sheaths and the multipolar mapping catheter that are subject to less movement during the ablation procedure [19].

Char may form on the electrodes of the ablation catheter if high temperatures are achieved at the electrode-tissue interface particularly when there is not sufficient cooling from the blood pool. An impedance rise during applications of RF energy may indicate development of char and should prompt withdrawal and inspection of the catheter tip. With the availability of ablation catheters that have a tip electrode with an open irrigation system, the risk of char formation appears to be significantly reduced.

Endocardial RFCA disrupts the endothelial integrity and may expose a nidus of interstitial tissue that may facilitate thrombus formation. To prevent TEs during dissolution of any thrombus that may form on the endocardial surface as fibrosis and endothelial repair occurs, it is critical to maintain adequate anticoagulation after the ablation procedure. Regardless of whether there are any preprocedural risk factors for TEs or whether AF had been paroxysmal or chronic, patients are typically anticoagulated with warfarin for 8–12 weeks after ablation with a target INR level of 2–2.5 unless higher INR values are desirable due to preexisting comorbid conditions. This approach will also minimize the risk of new thrombus formation that may develop due to left atrial mechanical stunning within first week after ablation.

Late postablation thromboembolic events

Although restoration and maintenance of sinus rhythm by catheter ablation may be expected to eliminate the risk of late TEs in patients with AF, the effect of ablation on TE risk may be more than just control of AF. It is possible that patients with AF may have comorbid conditions that may predispose to TEs regardless of whether sinus rhythm is maintained or not [20,21]. Patients with CHADS$_2$ scores ≥ 2 are five times more likely to experience a TE when compared with those with a score of 0 [22,23].

Nevertheless, there are three observational reports from two large single center and one multicenter experience involving over 4000 patients that suggest that patients without recurrent AF based on ECG monitoring after AF ablation and the absence of recurrent symptoms may be of sufficient low risk even with a CHADS$_2$ score ≥ 2 that anticoagulation with warfarin may be stopped [24–26]. These data are encouraging and although not strong enough evidence to establish new guidelines for anticoagulation use, clearly suggest that therapy should be individualized and furthermore identify the need for a larger scale prospective, randomized study to confirm the ability to identify a low-risk group after successful AF ablation.

Strategies to prevent thromboembolic events (see also Chapter 6)

(i) Prior to AF ablation procedure: To minimize the risk of TEs, a TEE is often performed to rule out intracardiac thrombus particularly in patients with chronic AF, and also in patients with paroxysmal AF who may have additional risk factors such as prior stroke, marked left atrial dilatation, etc. The role of routine TEE in patients with paroxysmal AF at low risk for TEs has been less clear and varies from one center to the other. ICE has been increasingly used during AF ablation. It may be possible to visualize the LAA by ICE although intracardiac imaging has been shown to be less sensitive when compared with TEE in one study [27].

Although there may be variations in preoperative anticoagulation regimens among various centers, a common approach has been to discontinue warfarin 3–4 days prior to the ablation procedure and use LMWH at full dose until the night before the procedure. In patients who have not been on warfarin prior to the procedure, routine preoperative anticoagulation is often not necessary. However, routine anticoagulation for 2–3 months prior to the ablation procedure has also been performed in some centers.

In a recent multicenter study [28], 6454 patients were separated into 3 co-horts: group 1, underwent AF ablation with an 8-mm catheter off warfarin; group 2, underwent AF ablation with an open irrigated catheter off warfarin; group 3 underwent AF ablation with an open irrigated catheter during therapeutic anticoagulation with warfarin. Periprocedural stroke or TIA occurred in 27 patients (1.1%) in group 1 and 12 patients (0.9%) in group 2. Despite a higher prevalence of chronic AF and increased number of patients with $CHADS_2$ scores >2, no stroke or TIA was reported in group 3. Other studies have shown no difference in outcomes of cardiac tamponade in patients who underwent AF ablation procedures under therapeutic anticoagulation with warfarin [16].

(ii) During AF ablation procedure: As soon as or even prior to the TSP, systemic anticoagulation should be started with an intravenous bolus of heparin (usually 100 U/kg). Although different values of ACT have been targeted in various laboratories, an ACT of 300–350 seconds is usually adequate [36]. ICE identified thrombus appears be more common when spontaneous echo contrast has been observed, or if severe left atrial enlargement is present with target ACT above 350 seconds demonstrated to prevent such thrombi even in high-risk patients [29]. ACT should be checked every 20–30 minutes throughout the procedure. Target ACT levels can be maintained by either intermittent additional boluses of heparin or continuous infusion of heparin usually at 1000–2000 U/h. Systemic anticoagulation just prior to the TSP (after confirming the needle position with ICE) has also been utilized to minimize the risk of thrombus formation. Ablation should not be started without achieving adequate anticoagulation. After catheters and sheaths are removed from the LA, systemic anticoagulation can be discontinued. Sheaths often can be removed safely once ACT < 180 seconds. Caution should be deployed when using protamine to reverse the therapeutic effects of heparin as it may be associated with allergic reactions and hypotension particularly in diabetic patients. Concern for increased thrombogenicity with protamine and the requirement for higher doses of heparin when reinitiating anticoagulation after the sheath removal has tempered its routine use. Some centers use a low dose of protamine when ACT is very elevated at the end of the procedure (>300 seconds) to partially reverse anticoagulation and facilitate sheath removal. The risk of an allergic reaction is not eliminated by such low dose administration. Of note, allergic reactions with protamine are characteristically associated with profound increases in pulmonary artery pressure, which may be persistent and may require aggressive supportive measures to prevent homodynamic collapse.

(iii) After AF ablation: An approach to anticoagulation after AF ablation has been to restart heparin infusion without a bolus 4 hours after the sheath removal if AF ablation was not performed with a therapeutic INR. Heparin infusion is often maintained until the next morning during an overnight hospital stay. Warfarin should be started at the regular maintenance dose the same day. Using a higher loading dose may actually have a prothrombotic effect.

To shorten the hospital stay, patients may be discharged home on half dose LMWH the day after the ablation. LMWH should be administered until the INR becomes therapeutic (>2.0). All patients should be anticoagulated with warfarin for 12 weeks after ablation with a target INR level of 2–3.0. Routine use of antiplatelet agents in addition to warfarin after AF ablation does not appear to be associated with a decrease in the risk of TEs [30]; however, increase in peripheral vascular complications have been noted [3].

As maintaining therapeutic anticoagulation with warfarin during AF ablation becomes more widely adopted, there will be no need for additional heparin administration after the procedure. It should be noted that the majority of perioperative TEs occur within the first week after the ablation, when anticoagulation can be suboptimal due to bridging with LMWH and reinitiating warfarin. Therefore, maintaining therapeutic anticoagulation with warfarin during LARFA may reduce the incidence of early perioperative TEs.

Dabigatran, a direct oral thrombin inhibitor, has recently become available for anticoagulation. Dabigatran does not require monitoring of anticoagulation, therapeutic anticoagulation is achieved usually within few hours, and is not subject to dietary interactions. Despite its cost, twice daily dosing, and potential for gastrointestinal side effects, dabigatran is likely to be used for anticoagulation in many patients with AF [31]. The utility of dabigatran for periprocedural anticoagulation has not been studied. Two potential areas of concern are the lack of a specific antidote to reverse the anticoagulant effects in case of an emergency, such as major bleeding, and inability to determine patient compliance and whether therapeutic anticoagulation has been achieved prior to the procedure. Although ecarin clotting time can be used to determine the anticoagulant effect, this test may not be widely available. However, dabigatran may more readily be used for postprocedural anticoagulation in patients who undergo LARFA after having discontinued oral anticoagulants prior to the procedure, and it is likely to shorten the duration of bridging with LMWH as therapeutic levels are achieved within few hours of administration.

PV stenosis

PV stenosis is a new clinical entity specifically related to RF catheter ablation of AF [32,33]. The incidence was reported to be up to 40% when ablation targeted focal triggers inside the PVs [34,35]. With the evolution of PVI techniques and ablation at the vein ostium or even more proximal to the venoatrial junction, the incidence of severe stenosis has decreased to 0.5–2% [7,36–39]. However, PV stenosis may be underreported because most of the patients remain asymptomatic. In the updated worldwide registry, the rate of PV stenosis requiring intervention was 0.29% [1]. To reduce the risk of PV stenosis when RF ablation is performed near the PV ostium, the anatomy should be clearly defined. To localize the PV ostium and to avoid ablation inside the vein, angiography of the PVs, ICE, 3D mapping systems eventually with integration of MR or CT imaging anatomic information and impedance measurements using the ablation catheter has been used [40–43]. Whatever monitoring/imaging technique is used, the decisive factor in avoiding PV stenosis seems to be a fundamental understanding of the anatomy of the LA, coupled with the ability to identify the location of lesion deployment. Avoidance of lesion placement within venous structure is critical [44]. At selected sites such as the anterior margin of the left-sided veins that abuts the LA appendage or the carina between ipsilateral veins, titration of energy delivery may avoid excessive tissue disruption and subsequent narrowing. Cryoenergy was promoted to eliminate the risk of PV stenosis. In a prospective study including 346 patients, no PV stenosis was found using the cryoballoon technique for PVI [45]. However, the first cases of PV stenosis after cryoballoon PVI have been reported recently [46,47]. Randomized trials comparing RF energy with the cryoballoon and other new tools for PVI such as the multielectrode-phased RF ablation catheter (PVAC) will be necessary to establish the real rate of PV stenosis with each technology.

The clinical manifestation of PV stenosis may be quite insidious. Many people are asymptomatic if only single vein stenosis is present [35]. Symptoms will depend on the number of stenotic veins, the degree of stenosis, and the time course of stenosis [40,44,48,49]. The most frequent symptoms of PV stenosis are cough, dyspnea, hemoptysis, or recurrent and drug-resistant pneumonia [40,44,48]. Symptoms may develop both early and/or late after the procedure with most patients presenting within 2–6 months [44]. To diagnose PV stenosis, TEE and ICE including Doppler measurements [50], V/Q lung scan [40,44], MR [51] or CT imaging [44] may be used (Figures 7.1 and 7.2).

Significant (>70%) PV stenosis in symptomatic patients should be treated by angioplasty and/or stenting [52]. Angioplasty is associated with high restenosis rate of 45% [43,52]. PV stenting with bare metal stents with a size of ≥10 mm [53,54] or drug-eluting stents [55] seem to reduce the restenosis rate. Surgical interventions may be considered, but because of the disappointing surgical results for congenital stenosis, surgery should be considered the treatment of last resort. In asymptomatic patients with two or more stenosed PVs, invasive therapy might be considered to prevent pulmonary hypertension during exercise [56]. Whether patients with one stenosed PV and no or minimal clinical symptoms should be treated is not yet known. Regression as well as progression of PV stenosis to complete occlusion has been observed during follow-up [33,51]. Anticoagulation is typically maintained if severe stenosis is present to prevent acute thrombosis.

PN injury

The right PN has a close anatomic relationship with the RSPV and SVC as it runs along the lateral and posterolateral wall of the RA and anterior to the RSPV. The right PN is vulnerable to collateral injury during endocardial RF

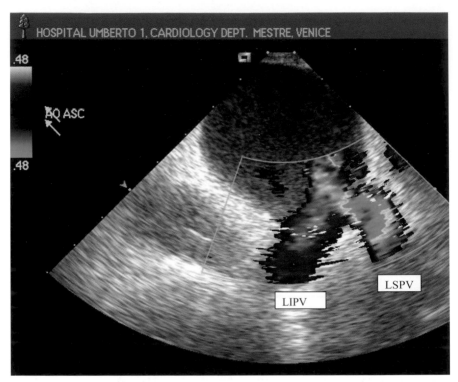

Figure 7.1 Intracardiac echocardiogram with color-Doppler measurement of flow velocity in the LIPV and LSPV in a patient during a redo procedure, 6 months after a first AF ablation. The flow velocity is increased with aliasing effect in the LSPV as expression of mild-to-moderate postablation PV stenosis.

delivery at or close to these structures [57–62] (Figure 7.3). As more extensive ablation procedures are performed for persistent AF, the left PN can also be susceptible to injury when RF lesions are applied in the vicinity of the LAA [63].

Experimental evidence has shown that the PN may be particularly susceptible to thermal injury [59]. Permanent nerve damage may be preceded by transitory loss of function, opening a window for early recognition and prevention by close monitoring. Locating the right PN before ablation can also help in predicting risk and preventing injury. Imaging the right pericardiophrenic artery with CT angiography before the procedure can reliably locate the PN and help identifying vulnerable anatomy [64].

Bai et al. [65] reported 16 cases of right PN injury (81% during AF ablation and 19% during sinus node modification), with an estimated incidence around 0.1%. Most patients (88%) had persistent nerve damage, with only 2 presenting with transient loss of function. Nonetheless, recovery was documented in all cases after a mean of 7.6 months of follow-up (range 3–28 months).

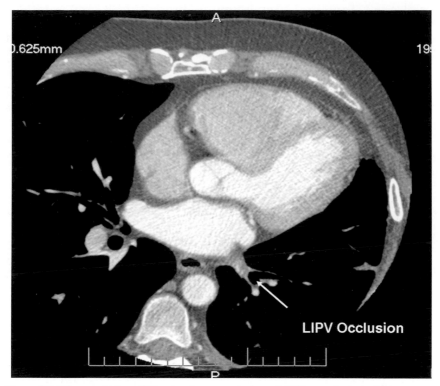

Figure 7.2 CT scan of LA and PVs, showing an occlusion of LIPV in a patient who had undergone AF ablation 3 months before.

Sacher et al. [66] reported 18 patients with PN injury during AF ablation of 3755 consecutive patients (prevalence of 0.48%). Interestingly, two cases of left PN injury occurred during ablation of non-PV foci at the LA appendage roof (Figure 7.3). The remaining cases presented with right PN injury attributable to ablation lesions at the inferoanterior region of the RSPV or the posterolateral SVC. Complete recovery was documented in 66% after a mean of 4.5 months after the index procedure. Partial recovery occurred in an additional 17% after 36 months of follow-up. PN injury appears to be clinically silent in the majority of cases, although symptoms may also depend on the previous existing lung function. In fact, in the above-mentioned series 50% [65] and 22% [66] were completely asymptomatic, with the majority of the remaining patients presenting with mild symptoms such as dyspnea, cough, and weakness. However, some patients developed more severe lung complications such as pneumonia, atelectasis, pleural effusion, and respiratory failure requiring mechanical support. One patient with persistent dyspnea required surgical plication of the paralyzed right diaphragm.

The diagnosis of PN injury can be confirmed by fluoroscopy demonstrating a positive "sniff test" and the presence of unilateral diaphragmatic paralysis

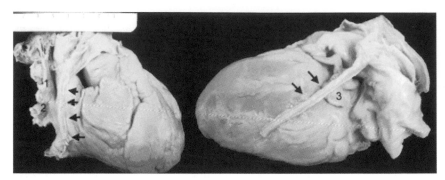

Figure 7.3 Anatomic relationships between right PN and heart (left) and left PN and heart (right):
1, RSPV; 2, RIPV; 3, LAA. (Reproduced from Sacher F, Monahan KH, Thomas SP, et al. Phrenic
nerve injury after atrial fibrillation catheter ablation: characterization and outcome in a multicenter
study. J Am Coll Cardiol 2006; 47:2498–2503.)

(Figure 7.4). It is important to note that catheter-induced PN injury has been
observed with the use of different energy sources [65–74], including balloon
ultrasound, laser, RF, and even cryoablation.

Despite the low prevalence and apparent benign course in most patients,
prevention of persistent PN injury is possible by identification of PN location with high-output pacing and avoiding energy application in these regions [59,65,66]. Such high-output pacing (≥30 mA, 2 ms) is recommended
before energy delivery at or near the RSPV, the SVC, and the proximal LA appendage roof and, in the case of diaphragmatic contraction, ablation should be
avoided. Other methods have recently been reported to allow RF delivery in
regions where PN injury would be expected. Applying a intrapericardial balloon [75,76] and progressive infusion of air and saline in the pericardial space
in a controlled fashion [77] to separate the PN from the epicardial surface has

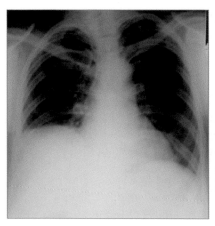
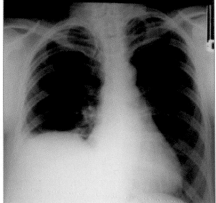

Figure 7.4 Chest X-ray just after AF ablation, showing right unilateral diaphragmatic paralysis as
a consequence of right PN injury during the procedure.

been performed by experienced operators, allowing successful ablation where PN injury would otherwise occur. Another option, though less validated and with greater inherent risk because dysfunction is already identified, includes close monitoring of the diaphragmatic excursion with immediate offset of ablation upon its reduction or if hiccups develop.

Atrioesophageal fistula

Atrioesophageal fistulas, esophageal damage, and perforation were first described following RF ablation on the posterior wall of the LA during open-heart surgery in 2001. Ablation was performed endocardially with patients on cardiopulmonary bypass. Patients presented with neurological deficits from air emboli, massive gastrointestinal bleeding, and septic shock on postoperative days 5–7 [78,79]. In 2004, the first descriptions of atrioesophageal fistula formation following percutaneous RF catheter ablation were published [80,81] (Figure 7.5). The patients in the published cases presented with nonspecific signs and symptoms including dysphagia, odynophagia, intermittent cardiac or neurological ischemia (air emboli and/or vegetations), persistent fever, bacteremia, fungemia, and melena [82]. The mean reported time to presentation is 12.3 days [82] but recently has been described as late as 41 days following the procedure [83]. Although atrioesophageal fistula formation is apparently rare, it appears to be nearly universally fatal, and thus it has remained the subject of intense investigation. A nationwide survey of practicing electrophysiologists reported an incidence of 6 cases in 20,425 left atrial procedures (0.03%) with 5 deaths [84]. Evaluation of serial CT scans as well as ICE has documented the close proximity, often <0.5 cm, of the esophagus to the left atrial wall [85–87] (Figure 7.6). Some laboratories have also documented movement of the

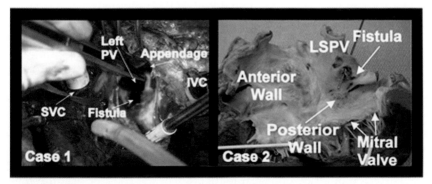

Figure 7.5 Postmortem anatomic specimen of a patient who died after having developed an atrioesophageal fistula after an AF ablation procedure. The LA was incised near the LSPV and opened in book fashion, with anterior wall on left and posterior wall on right. Probe passes through fistula, which was on posterior wall near LSPV. (Reproduced from Pappone C, Oral H, Santinelli V, et al. Atrio-esophageal fistula as a complication of percutaneous transcatheter ablation of atrial fibrillation. Circulation 2004; 109:2724–2726.)

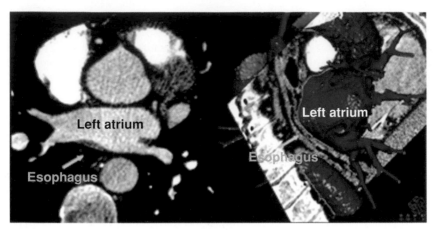

Figure 7.6 Three-dimensional computed tomographic reconstruction of the LA in relation to the esophagus. (Reproduced from Cummings JE, Schweikert RA, Saliba WI, et al. Brief communication: atrial-esophageal fistulas after radiofrequency ablation. Ann Intern Med 2006;144:572–574, with permission from Annals of Internal Medicine.)

esophagus during an ablation procedure [88]. Three-dimensional mapping systems including Carto and EnSite, the ingestion of radiopaque contrast, and online ICE have all been used to image the esophagus before, during, and following ablation [87]. Injury to the esophagus is presumed to be thermal in nature. Endoscopically visible ulcerations have been demonstrated in 1.6% of patients on the day following ablation [89–91], although most do not progress to fistula formation. While some may argue that ablation in the region of the posterior LA wall is not safe and should be avoided, others believe that monitoring of esophageal location and/or temperature and avoidance of overheating the endocardial surface (microbubble formation) and/or low-energy delivery for short duration offer safe options [85]. Because of the infrequent occurrence of atrioesophageal fistula, there are currently no data that clearly places one approach superior to another although esophageal fistula has been reported in patients in whom RF delivery was dictated by temperature monitoring. Damage to the esophagus has been also documented following AF ablation using robotic navigation. Data, thus far, clearly demonstrate that atrioesophageal fistula is characteristically a fatal complication [82,84]. Surgical intervention to prevent fatality requires rapid and accurate recognition and diagnosis. Fever, malaise, leukocytosis, dysphagia, hematemesis, and neurological symptoms in patients with a recent catheter ablation procedure should raise suspicion of atrioesophageal fistula. CT of the chest or head revealing intravascular air should immediately suggest a communication between the gastrointestinal tract and the vasculature. Currently, imaging techniques such as MR or CT are recommended to diagnose an atrioesophageal fistula. If a fistula is suspected, it is important that endoscopy is avoided because insufflation of the esophagus has been demonstrated to lead to massive air emboli through the fistula leading to stroke and myocardial infarction [78–82]. Although mortality of this complication is very high, previously published reports documented survival following rapid surgical correction [80]. Stenting of the esophagus has also been reported to be effective [90].

Periesophageal vagal injury

An unusual extracardiac complication of AF ablation characterized by abdominal bloating and discomfort occurring within a few hours to 2 days after the procedure has been described [92]. The incidence of such adverse event was 1% in a series of 367 patients. This complication is probably due to LA RF energy delivery affecting the periesophageal vagal plexus. Upper gastrointestinal investigation showed a pyloric spasm, gastric hypomotility, and a markedly prolonged gastric emptying time. To avoid this complication, the authors suggested using esophageal temperature monitoring and avoiding LA endocardium overlying the esophagus. Moreover, identification of the esophageal vagal plexus and the titration of power according to the myocardial thickness and surrounding structures should be helpful.

Vascular complications

Among the most common complications of AF ablation are vascular complications including femoral arteriovenous fistula, pseudoaneurysm, and large hematomas. These groin complications are due to the numerous vascular access sites required for the procedure and high-intensity anticoagulation during and following the procedure. The prevalence of pseudoaneurysm ranges from 0.15–0.93% and 0.3–1.3% for AV fistula in large series [1–4,7]. Suggestions for preventing vascular complications include use of smaller gauge needles for venous access, avoid femoral arterial access, perform procedure on warfarin anticoagulation to avoid the need for parenteral "bridging" anticoagulation [93]. Other suggestions include decreasing number of sheaths in one vein, use of micropuncture kits, and use of ultrasound guided access. Treatment of pseudoaneurysm depends on the size and complexity and can include surgical repair but most are treated with ultrasound guided compression and thrombin injection [94,95]. Treatment of AV fistula is also dependent on the size and complexity and includes simple observation, ultrasound guided compression, endovascular stent and surgery, but most can be treated with simple observation. In one large study of vascular complication postinterventional cardiology procedures, only 11% of AV fistulas required surgical repair with the vast majority able to be treated conservatively [96].

Acute coronary artery injury

Based on the success of the surgical maze procedure, linear lesions are frequently deployed to improve efficacy of ablative therapy. In a postmortem analysis, Wittkampf et al. [97] described that RF applications on the distal portion of the mitral isthmus could create coronary circumflex injury, given the fact that a distance of <5 mm from the endocardium exists in about 30% of the population. Fortunately, coronary injury is an uncommon complication but can be fatal [11]. Takahashi et al. described an incidence of 0.002% of clinically evident circumflex artery occlusion in a large series of patients who underwent mitral isthmus ablation. In 71% of the study group, RF energy was delivered in the CS [98]. To avoid this complication, a more posterior mitral isthmus line could be chosen, but it is possible that other anatomic structures could have strong relationships with the posterior wall of the LA. Assessing the location of the circumflex coronary vessel and its proximity to the planned ablation sites should be considered with careful power titration as appropriate. Concern about subclinical but permanent damage to the coronary that may lead to late stenosis requires additional investigation.

Air emboli

Air emboli may enter the arterial system during TSP, sheath/catheter exchanges, aspiration, irrigation, intravenous medication administration, or continuous infusion of sheaths [99–101]. An air embolus often travels to the right coronary artery and mimics typical clinical presentations of acute inferior myocardial wall ischemia. If the procedure is performed under conscious sedation, the patient may complain of chest pain. There may also be ST elevation in the inferior ECG leads. Air embolus to the coronary arteries often resolves within several minutes without major complications and residual myocardial injury, although hypotension and acute myocardial dysfunction may be profound and aggressive supportive measures may be required. If the signs suggestive of an embolus persist, coronary angiography and, if necessary, aspiration of the air from within the coronary artery should be considered. Air emboli may also travel to cerebral circulation and may lead to severe neurological manifestations. Treatment of large air emboli with prompt hyperbaric oxygen may have clinical value [102]. Air emboli are best prevented by proper attention to catheter and sheath technique. Caution should be exercised when exchanging the sheaths and catheters. The sheaths should routinely be flushed intermittently and also after each catheter withdrawal. Air filters can be used to minimize the risk of a large air embolus. If sheaths are continuously irrigated throughout the procedure, automatic pumps capable of detecting air in the tubing should be considered.

Catheter entrapment in the MV or PV

The original worldwide survey on AF ablation on 7154 patients reported an incidence of 0.01% of valve damage because of catheter entrapment in the MV apparatus [7]. The CMC is at particular risk for entrapment within the mitral apparatus [103]. Several recommendations can be made to reduce the incidence of such a complication. First, an effort should be made to always position the circular part of the mapping catheter in the posterior LA during transseptal catheterization. Second, it is recommended to torque the catheter in a clockwise direction when leaving the transseptal sheath in order to avoid the tip of the catheter from becoming entrapped in anatomic structures that have a diameter less than that of the CMC. These first two tips have allowed for safe catheter manipulation and successful ablation even in the setting of prior mitral surgery and prosthetic MV [104,105]. Third, it is recommended to advance the catheter and/or the sheath over the catheter when such entrapment is observed. This may prevent a further tightening of the catheter loop and frequently frees up the tangled apparatus [106]. Finally, early surgical extraction, which carries a small but unknown risk of thromboembolization, should be strongly considered before manual extraction in order to avoid MV injury and preserve the MV apparatus [107]. Rarely the CMC can get entrapped in the PV with the potential risk of laceration and intrapulmonary bleeding [108].

Organized left atrial tachyarrhythmias after AF ablation

Organized left atrial tachycardias and flutter are common in patients who have undergone left AF ablation with a reported incidence of 1.2 to 40% [109–128] (Table 7.3). The variability in the frequency of occurrence postablation and the mechanism of the tachycardia appears to be clearly dependent on the type of ablation procedure used and the extent of the underlying atrial disease [126,127,130,131,133]. Centers utilizing circumferential PV ablation combined with additional linear lesions in the LA, targeting of fractionated electrograms and other more extensive LA ablation report a higher prevalence of macroreentrant atypical flutters and an overall incidence of organized LA tachycardias that is more than 5–10X that observed with only PVI procedures or limited atrial ablation of non-PV triggers [109–131]. This is especially true if no attempt is made to establish/confirm a line of bidirectional block or anchor clusters of more extensive LA ablation to anatomic obstacles [115,132,133]. Since more extensive left atrial ablation beyond PVI are typically applied to patients with more persistent forms of AF, the incidence of LA flutter post more extensive ablation is greater in this patient population [130].

The macroreentrant circuit of atypical flutter typically moves around a large anatomic barrier such as the mitral annulus or ipsilateral PVs and typically incorporates a zone of slow conduction created by gaps in LA linear lesions [134,135]. Occasionally, circuits can be defined around the fossa ovalis, originate from the CS musculature and adjacent LA, or involve smaller circuits around anatomic barriers related to prior surgical or catheter based lesions [136,137]. Centers that utilize PVI alone have observed a low overall incidence of recurrent regular atrial tachycardias, and these arrhythmias have been predominantly localized reentrant LA tachycardias originating from reconnected PVs [112,113,123,131,138].

Table 7.3 Iatrogenic postatrial fibrillation ablation LAT/FL: literature data.

Author	Number of patients	LAT/FL (%)	Time to LAT/FL (mo)	Mean TCL (ms)	Macroreentry	Focus	Acute success (%)	Chronic success (%)	Mean follow-up (mo)
Kanagaratnam et al. [118]	71	14 (20)	NR	NR	5/5[a]	0	100	100	NR
Villacastin et al. [120]	30	2 (6.6)	2	240	2	0	100	100	6.5
Oral et al. [119]	80	1 (1.2)	NR	NR	1	0	100	100	NR
Ernst et al. [121]	88	6 (7.0)	NR	NR	6	0	100	100	NR
Gerstenfeld et al. [131]	341	10 (3.4)	5.7 ± 2.8[b]	253 ± 33	1	8	100	100	6.7 ± 2.3
Mesas et al. [110]	276	13 (4.7)	2.6 ± 1.6[b]	275 ± 25	11	3	100	87	2.5 ± 1.2
Pappone et al. [115]	560	39 (7.0)[c]	2.4/2.9	NR	31	8	100	100	6.3/8.2
Jais et al. [117]	100	12 (12)	NR	NR	9	3	100	87[d]	12
Oral et al. [122]	100	21 (21)	NR	NR	NR	NR	NR	NR	NR
Ouyang et al. [113]	100	21 (21)	0.21	206	17	2	100	100	5.8 ± 1.8
Cummings et al. [123]	737	23 (3.1)	NR	NR	23	0	100	51	16.5 ± 2.9
Hocini et al. [124]	20	4 (20)	4 ± 1[b]	NR	4	0	100	100	NR
Chugh et al. [111]	349	85 (24)	1.5 ± 2.0	238 ± 35	28/28[a]	0	88	82	7.5 ± 4
Shah et al. [116]	207	16 (8)	2.3 ± 2.0	271 ± 45	15/15[a]	0	93	87	21 ± 11
Daoud et al. [125]	112	28 (25)	1.0 ± 0.5	NR	9/9[a]	0	94	NR	NR
Deisenhofer et al. [114]	67	21 (31)	3.2 ± 3.1	264 ± 41	16/16[a]	0	89	38	10.4 ± 6.7
Chae et al. [126]	800	78(10)	NR	256 ± 49	137/155	18/155	86	77	13 ± 10
Sawhney et al. [127]	66	8(12)	9.8 ± 4.9[b]	NR	9/9	0	100	83	NR
Rostock et al. [128]	320	128(40)	NR	270 ± 40	44/61[a]	17/61[a]	93	82	21 ± 4
Chang et al. [129]	452	87(19)	NR	NR	84/120	36/120	90	97	21 ± 16

Adapted from Raviele A, Themistoclakis S, Rossillo A, Bonso A. Iatrogenic postatrial fibrillation ablation left atrial tachycardia/flutter: How to prevent and treat it? J Cardiovasc Electrophysiol 2005; 16:298–301.

[a] Only a limited number of the total population of patients with LAT/FL underwent repeat ablation procedure.

[b] Time to LAT/FL ablation.

[c] 28 (10%) in the 280 patients who were randomized to circumferential ablation alone, and 11 (3.9%) in the 280 patients who were randomized to circumferential plus linear lesions ablation.

[d] Regards both AF and LAT/FL.

Most of the regular LA tachycardias that occur after ablation will be manifested early in the postablation course. Patients are frequently very symptomatic because they tend to demonstrate 2:1 AV conduction and a faster ventricular rate than observed in response to AF. Most of the tachycardias are also resistant to drug therapy. Despite the general poor response to medical therapy and frequent recurrence after cardioversion, attempts to temporize are still recommended when the arrhythmia is observed early postablation. This is especially true given the fact that up to 50% of these tachycardias appear to resolve spontaneously during the "healing phase" postablation [111]. Because many tachycardias will persist after the 2–3-month blanking period and/or are recurrent and very symptomatic, repeat ablation procedures are appropriate.

The 12-lead ECG may be helpful in suggesting a focal source for the LA tachycardia from a reconnected PV or macroreentry around the mitral annulus [127,131]. A superior and posterior location for the PV creates inferiorly directed P waves with a positive precordial activation pattern [139–141]. Importantly, right AFL and LA tachycardias that occur after extensive LA ablation can create atypical surface ECG patterns during the tachycardia [142]. The ability to identify accurately the origin/path of regular atrial tachycardias that occur after AF ablation is critically dependent on the use of detailed activation mapping primarily for focal atrial tachycardias and/or entrainment mapping techniques [116,126,131,143,144].

Depending on the underlying mechanism, the ablation strategy either may require isolation of the reconnected PV segment (for focal or local reentrant tachycardias of PV origin) or may involve targeting the zone of slow conduction or a well-defined anatomic isthmus for macroreentrant flutter [112,117,131]. It is routine to reisolate PVs even if the mechanism of the LA flutter is macroreentry to minimize the risk of manifest AF and recurrent LA flutter if lines of block do not hold long term [131]. Mitral annular lines can be especially difficult to create and bidirectional block frequently requires ablation within the CS to target the directly opposite endocardial ablation sites [97,131,145,146]. Care must be taken to avoid damage to the circumflex coronary vessel that may be in close proximity. Alternative anterior lines of block from the anterior mitral annulus to the superior PVs have been used when mitral annular lines with bidirectional block are difficult to create or when zones of slow conduction from LA disease or previous ablation lesions make these lines important to close gaps of slow conduction during mitral annular or figure of eight AFLs [147].

Overall, ablation is quite effective for these postablation LA tachycardias with reported long-term success in excess of 80%. The frequent occurrence of macroreentrant rhythms associated with LA linear lesions has made it imperative that this lesion strategy should only be used when felt to be clinically necessary. Most investigators consider the LA tachycardias to be a true proarrhythmic effect of more extensive LA catheter ablation rather than a transitional arrhythmia observed during attempts at eliminating AF [125,148]. As a result, linear ablation with roof and mitral annular lines and more extensive defragmentation are now less commonly performed in the setting of paroxysmal AF to minimize the risk of this complication. In addition, documentation of bidirectional block using the appropriate stimulation techniques is performed routinely when lines are created to attempt to minimize the chance that a proarrhythmic effect from slowing conduction without block has been created [115,132,133].

Adverse impact on atrial contractility

Reverse remodeling of the left cardiac chambers with improvement in function has been reported after successful RF catheter ablation of paroxysmal and persistent AF [149–154]. However, the consequences of RF ablation on the LA contractility are still somewhat inconsistent based on published reports.

A recent meta-analysis, including 17 studies and 869 patients, assessed the effect of RF catheter ablation on left atrial size, volume, and function in patients with AF. Independent of the technique applied there was a significant decrease in LA diameters and volumes during follow-up in those without AF recurrence but not in those with AF recurrence. LAEF and LA active emptying fraction did not decrease in patients without AF recurrence, whereas they decreased in patients with AF recurrence [149].

In PVI studies, there was no change in the LA active emptying fraction in patients with paroxysmal AF. Otherwise, an increase in active emptying fraction was observed in patients with chronic AF; the mean LAEF 1 day after ablation was $32 \pm 11\%$ compared with $54 \pm 18\%$ in the same patients at 6 months [150]. In patients undergoing cine electron-beam CT to assess LAEF, there was also a significant improvement in LAEF post-PVI from $17 \pm 6\%$ to $22 \pm 5\%$ ($p = .01$) [151]. In contrast, in a circumferential PV ablation study, patients undergoing LA contractile function evaluation by gated, multiphase, dynamic contrast enhanced CT scans showed that LAEF was lower after ablation ($21 \pm 8\%$ vs. $32 \pm 13\%$, $p = .003$). Furthermore, LAEF after catheter ablation was similar among patients with paroxysmal AF and those with chronic AF ($21 \pm 8\%$ vs. $23 \pm 13\%$, $p = .7$) and LAEF after catheter ablation was lower in all patients with AF than in control subjects ($21 \pm 10\%$ vs. $47 \pm 5\%$, $p < .001$) [21].

It appears that the effects of RF ablation on LA function are dependent on the extent of ablation and time it was assessed. Extensive ablation during PVAI causes initial impairment in atrial function; however, the positive remodeling that occurs with rhythm restoration in patients with a high burden of AF typically outweighs negative effects of ablation [153,154].

Finally, it is important to recognize that many studies have used different protocols to evaluate the LA size, included different patient populations, and incorporated different ablation techniques. Furthermore, currently there is no standardization in the measurement of LA function and the timing of its assessment. These limitations suggest that more investigation and standardization is still required in this important area.

Radiation exposure during catheter ablation of AF

Catheter ablation of AF frequently requires a long fluoroscopy time. Further complicating the issue is the fact that AF ablation procedures are often done in the obese patient increasing the exposure to patient and operator. Very low frame rate pulsed fluoroscopy systems have become the norm to minimize radiation exposure. Skin radiation "burns" with proper operating equipment are currently extremely rare [155,156]. Limiting cineangiography and avoidance of magnification are also suggested to reduce further radiation exposure. Changing the angulation of fluoroscopic equipment may help to further reduce direct skin exposure when prolonged procedure and imaging times are required. A carefully monitored and aggressive approach to minimize x-ray exposure can be successful in minimizing exposure [157,158].

Although single procedure exposure appears to represent a very low cancer risk, repeated procedures may indeed begin to produce a measurable risk increase and every effort should be made to minimize total exposure [159–161].

EAM with preprocedure left atrial image integration and remote navigation systems that facilitate catheter placement and stability appear to help reduce fluoroscopy exposure [162–165]. Operator exposure can also be reduced by use of appropriate lead shielding. More complete cabin-like lead shielding and ceiling suspended lead shielding may help keep the operator who receives daily fluoroscopy exposure protected while minimizing deleterious effect of chronic lead apron weight bearing [166–168].

References

1. Cappato R, Calkins H, Chen SA, et al. Updated worldwide survey on the methods, efficacy, and safety of catheter ablation for human atrial fibrillation. Circ Arrhythm Electrophysiol 2010; 3:32–38.
2. Dagres N, Hindricks G, Kottkamp H, et al. Complications of atrial fibrillation ablation in a high-volume center in 1,000 procedures: Still cause for concern? J Cardiovasc Electrophysiol 2009; 20: 1014–1019.
3. Baman TS, Jongnarangsin K, Chugh A, et al. Prevalence and predictors of complications of radiofrequency catheter ablation for atrial fibrillation. J Cardiovasc Electrophysiol 2011; 22:126–631.
4. Leong-Sit P, Zado E, Callans DJ, et al. Efficacy and risk of atrial fibrillation ablation before 45 years of age. Circ Arrhythm Electrophysiol 2010; 3:452–457.
5. Hindricks G. The multicentre European radiofrequency survey (MERFS): Complications of radiofrequency catheter ablation of arrhythmias. Eur Heart J 1993; 14:1644–1653.
6. Scheinman MM, Huang S. The 1998 NASPE prospective catheter ablation registry. PACE 2000; 23:1020–1028.

7. Cappato R, Calkins H, Chen SA, et al. Worldwide survey on the methods, efficacy, and safety of catheter ablation for human atrial fibrillation. Circulation 2005; 111:1100–1105.

8. Lee G, Sparks PB, Morton JB, et al. Low risk of major complications associated with pulmonary vein antral isolation for atrial fibrillation: Results of 500 consecutive ablation procedures in patients with low prevalence of structural heart disease from a single center. J Cardiovasc Electrophysiol 2011; 22:163–168.

9. Cheema A, Dong J, Dalal D, et al. Long-term safety and efficacy of circumferential ablation with pulmonary vein isolation. J Cardiovasc Electrophysiol 2006; 17:1080–1085.

10. Cappato R, Calkins H, Chen SA, et al. Prevalence and causes of fatal outcome in catheter ablation of atrial fibrillation. J Am Coll Cardiol 2009; 53:1798–1803.

11. Hargrove M, Marshall CB, Jahanjir S, Hinchion J. Emergency bypass post percutaneous atrial ablation: A case report. Perfusion 2010; 25:423–424.

12. Ren J-F, Marchlinski FE, Callans DJ, Herrmann HC. Clinical Utility of Acu-Nav diagnostic ultrasound catheter imaging during left heart radiofrequency ablation and transcatheter closure procedures. J Am Soc Echocardiogr 2002; 15:1301–1308.

13. De Ponti R, Cappato R, Curnis A, et al. Trans-septal catheterization in the electrophysiology laboratory. Data from a multicenter survey spanning 12 years. J Am Coll Cardiol 2006; 47:1037–1042.

14. Hsu LF, Jaïs P, Hocini M, et al. Incidence and prevention of cardiac tamponade complicating ablation for atrial fibrillation. Pacing Clin Electrophysiol 2005; 28:S106–S109.

15. Lambert T, Steinwender C, Leisch F, Hofmann R. Cardiac tamponade following pericarditis 18 days after catheter ablation. Clin Res Cardiol 2010; 99:595–597.

16. Latchmansetty R, Gautam S, Bhakta S, et al. Management and outcome of cardiac tamponade during atrial fibrillation ablation in the presence of therapeutic anticoagulation with warfarin. Heart Rhythm 2011; 8:805–808.

17. Bertaglia E, Zoppo F, Tondo C, et al. Early complications of pulmonary vein catheter ablation for atrial fibrillation: A multicenter prospective registry on procedural safety. Heart Rhythm 2007; 4:1265–1271.

18. Patel D, Mohanty P, Di Biase L, et al. Outcomes and complications of catheter ablation for atrial fibrillation in females. Heart Rhythm 2010; 7:167–172.

19. Ren JF, Marchlinski FE, Callans DJ. Left atrial thrombus associated with ablation for atrial fibrillation: Identification with intracardiac echocardiography. J Am Coll Cardiol 2004; 43:1861–1867.

20. Lip GY. Does atrial fibrillation confer a hypercoagulable state? Lancet 1995; 346:1313–1314.

21. Lemola K, Desjardins B, Sneider M, et al. Effect of left atrial circumferential ablation for atrial fibrillation on left atrial transport function. Heart Rhythm 2005; 2:923–928.

22. Risk factors for stroke and efficacy of antithrombotic therapy in atrial fibrillation. Analysis of pooled data from five randomized controlled trials. Arch Intern Med 1994; 154:1449–1457.

23. Gage BF, Waterman AD, Shannon W, Boechler M, Rich MW, Radford MJ. Validation of clinical classification schemes for predicting stroke: Results from the National Registry of Atrial Fibrillation. JAMA 2001; 285:2864–2870.

24. Oral H, Chugh A, Ozaydin M, et al. Risk of thromboembolic events after percutaneous left atrial radiofrequency ablation of atrial fibrillation. Circulation 2006; 114:759–765.

25. Themistoclakis S, Corrado A, Marchlinski FE, et al. The risk of thromboembolism and need for oral anticoagulation after successful atrial fibrillation ablation. J Am Coll Cardiol 2010; 55:735–743.

26. Nademanee K, Schwab MC, Kosar EM, et al. Clinical outcomes of catheter substrate ablation for high-risk patients with atrial fibrillation. J Am Coll Cardiol 2008; 51:843–849.

27. Saksena S, Sra J, Jordaens L, et al. A prospective comparison of cardiac imaging using intracardiac echocardiography with transesophageal echocardiography in patients with atrial fibrillation. The intracardiac echocardiography guided cardioversion helps interventional procedures study. Circ Arrhythm Electrophysiol 2010; 3:571–577.

28. Di Biase L, Burkhardt JD, Mohanty P, et al. Periprocedural stroke and management of major bleeding complications in patients undergoing catheter ablation of atrial fibrillation: The impact of periprocedural therapeutic international normalized ratio. Circulation 2010; 121:2550–2556.

29. Ren JF, Marchlinski FE, Callans DJ, et al. Increased intensity of anticoagulation may reduce risk of thrombus during atrial fibrillation ablation procedures in patients with spontaneous echo contrast. J Cardiovasc Electrophysiol 2005; 16:474–477.

30. Wazni OM, Rossillo A, Marrouche NF, et al. Embolic events and char formation during pulmonary vein isolation in patients with atrial fibrillation: Impact of different anticoagulation regimens and importance of intracardiac echo imaging. J Cardiovasc Electrophysiol 2005; 16:576–581.

31. Connolly SJ, Ezekowitz MD, Yusuf S, et al.; RE-LY Steering Committee and Investigators. Dabigatran versus warfarin in patients with atrial fibrillation. N Engl J Med 2009; 361:1139–1151.

32. Robbins IM, Colvin EV, Doyle TP, et al. Pulmonary vein stenosis after catheter ablation of atrial fibrillation. Circulation 1998; 98:1769–1775.

33. Taylor GW, Kay GN, Zheng X, Bishop S, Idecker RE. Pathological effects of extensive radiofrequency energy application in the pulmonary veins in dogs. Circulation 2000; 101:1736–1742.

34. Yu WC, Hsu TL, Tai CT, et al. Acquired pulmonary vein stenosis after radiofrequency catheter ablation of paroxysmal atrial fibrillation. J Cardiovasc Electrophysiol 2001; 12:887–892.

35. Arentz T, Jander N, von Rosenthal J, et al. Incidence of pulmonary vein stenosis 2 years after radiofrequency catheter ablation of refractory atrial fibrillation. Eur Heart J 2003; 24:963–969.

36. Pappone C, Oreto G, Rosanio S, et al. Atrial electroanatomic remodeling after circumferential radiofrequency pulmonary vein ablation: Efficacy of an anatomic approach in a large cohort of patients with atrial fibrillation. Circulation 2001; 104:2539–2544.

37. Haissaguerre M, Shah DC, Jais P, et al. Electrophysiological breakthroughs from the left atrium to the pulmonary veins. Circulation 2000; 102:2463–2465.

38. Pappone C, Rosanio S, Oreto G, et al. Circumferential radiofrequency ablation of pulmonary vein ostia: A new anatomic approach for curing atrial fibrillation. Circulation 2000; 102:2619–2628.

39. Haissaguerre M, Jais P, Shah D, et al. Electrophysiological endpoint for catheter ablation of atrial fibrillation initiated from multiple pulmonary vein foci. Circulation 2000; 101:1409–1417.

40. Saad EB, Rossillo A, Saad CP, et al. Pulmonary vein stenosis after radiofrequency ablation of atrial fibrillation. Functional characterization, evolution, and influence of the ablation strategy. Circulation 2003; 108:3102–3107.

41. Kistler PM, Early MJ, Harris S, et al. Validation of three-dimensional cardiac image integration: Use of integrated CT image into electroanatomical mapping system to perform catheter ablation of atrial fibrillation. J Cardiovasc Electrophysiol 2006; 17:341–348.

42. Lang CC, Gugliotto F, Santinelli V, et al. Endocardial impedance mapping during circumferential pulmonary vein ablation of atrial fibrillation differentiates between atrial and venous tissue. Heart Rhythm 2006; 3:171–178.

43. Ren J-F, Marchlinski FE, Callans DJ, Zado ES. Intracardiac Doppler echocardiographic quantification of pulmonary vein flow velocity: An effective technique for monitoring pulmonary vein ostia narrowing during focal atrial fibrillation ablation. J Cardiovasc Electrophysiol 2002; 13:1076–1081.

44. Packer DL, Keelan P, Munger TM, et al. Clinical presentation, investigation, and management of pulmonary vein stenosis complicating ablation for atrial fibrillation. Circulation 2005; 111:546–554.

45. Neumann T, Vogt J, Schumacher B, et al. Circumferential pulmonary vein isolation with the cryoballoon technique: Results from a prospective 3-center study. J Am Coll Cardiol 2008; 52:273–278.

46. Cleland G, Poletta AP, Buga L, Ahmed D, Clark AL. Clinical trials update from American College of Cardiology meeting 2010: DOSE, ASPIRE, CONNECT, SPICH, STOP-AF, CABANA, RACE II, EVEREST II, ACCORD and NAVIGATOR. Eur J Heart Fail 2010; 12:623–629.

47. Thomas D, Katus HA, Voss F. Asymptomatic pulmonary vein stenosis after cryoballoon catheter ablation of paroxysmal atrial fibrillation. J Electrocardiol 2011; 44:473–476.

48. Di Biase L, Fahmy TS, Wazni, et al. Pulmonary vein total occlusion following catheter ablation for atrial fibrillation: clinical implications after long-term follow-up. J Am Coll Cardiol 2006; 48:2493–9.

49. Holmes DR, Monahan KH, Packer D. Pulmonary vein stenosis complicating ablation for atrial fibrillation. Clinical spectrum and interventional considerations. JACC Cardiovasc Interv 2009; 2:267–276.

50. Jander N, Minners J, Arentz T, et al. Transesophageal echocardiography in comparison with magnetic resonance imaging in the diagnosis of pulmonary vein stenosis after radiofrequency ablation therapy. J Am Soc Echocardiogr 2005; 18:654–659.

51. Dill T, Neumann T, Ekinci O, et al. Pulmonary vein diameter reduction after radiofrequency catheter ablation for paroxysmal atrial fibrillation evaluated by contrast enhanced three-dimensional magnetic resonance imaging. Circulation 2003; 107:845–850.

52. Quereshi AM, Prieto LR, Latson LA, et al. Transcatheter angioplasty for acquired pulmonary vein stenosis after radiofrequency ablation. Circulation 2003; 108:1336–1343.

53. Prieto LR, Schoenhagen P, Arruda MJ, et al. Comparison of stent versus balloon angioplasty for pulmonary vein stenosis complicating pulmonary vein isolation. J Cardiovasc Electrophysiol 2008; 19:673–678.

54. Neumann T, Kuniss M, Conradi G, et al. Pulmonary vein stenting for the treatment of acquired severe stenosis after pulmonary vein isolation. Clinical implications after long-term follow-up of 4 years. J Cardiovasc Electrophysiol 2009; 20:251–257.

55. De Potter TJ, Schmidt B, Chun KR, et al. Drug eluting stents for the treatment of pulmonary vein stenosis after atrial fibrillation ablation. Europace 2011; 13:57–61.

56. Arentz T, Weber R, Jander N, et al. Pulmonary hemodynamics at rest and during exercise in patients with significant pulmonary vein stenosis after radiofrequency catheter ablation for drug resistant atrial fibrillation. Eur Heart J 2005; 26:1410–1414.

57. Sanchez-Quintana D, Cabrera JA, Climent V, Farre J, Weiglein A, Ho SY. How close are the phrenic nerves to cardiac structures? Implications for cardiac interventionalists. J Cardiovasc Electrophysiol 2005; 16:309–313.

58. Fell SC. Surgical anatomy of the diaphragm and the phrenic nerve. Chest Surg Clin-NAm 1998; 8:281–294.
59. Bunch TJ, Bruce GK, Mahapatra S, et al. Mechanisms of phrenic nerve injury during radiofrequency ablation at the pulmonary vein orifice. J Cardiovasc Electrophysiol 2005; 16:1318–1325.
60. Lee BK, Choi KJ, Kim J, Rhee KS, Nam GB, Kim YH. Right phrenic nerve injury following electrical disconnection of the right superior pulmonary vein. Pacing Clin Electrophysiol 2004; 27:1444–1446.
61. Durante-Mangoni E, Del Vecchio D, Ruggiero G. Right diaphragm paralysis following cardiac radiofrequency catheter ablation for inappropriate sinus tachycardia. Pacing Clin Electrophysiol 2003; 26:783–784.
62. Lachman N, Syed FF, Habib A, et al. Correlative anatomy for the electrophysiologist, part ii: Cardiac ganglia, phrenic nerve, coronary venous system. J Cardiovasc Electrophysiol 2011; 22:104–110.
63. Sanchez-Quintana D, Ho SY, Climent V, Murillo M, Cabrera JA. Anatomic evaluation of the left phrenic nerve relevant to epicardial and endocardial catheter ablation: Implications for phrenic nerve injury. Heart Rhythm 2009; 6:764–768.
64. Horton R, Di Biase L, Reddy V, et al. Locating the right phrenic nerve by imaging the right pericardiophrenic artery with computerized tomographic angiography: Implications for balloon-based procedures. Heart Rhythm 2010; 7:937–941.
65. Bai R, Patel D, Di Biase L, et al. Phrenic nerve injury after catheter ablation: Should we worry about this complication? J Cardiovasc Electrophysiol 2006; 17:944–948.
66. Sacher F, Monahan KH, Thomas SP, et al. Phrenic nerve injury after atrial fibrillation catheter ablation: Characterization and outcome in a multicenter study. J Am Coll Cardiol 2006; 47:2498–2503.
67. Cummings JE, Pacifico A, Drago JL, Kilicaslan F, Natale A. Alternative energy sources for the ablation of arrhythmias. Pacing Clin Electrophysiol 2005; 28:434–443.
68. Antz M, Chun KJ, Ouyang F, Kuck KH. Ablation of atrial fibrillation in humans using a balloon-based ablation system: Identification of the site of phrenic nerve damage using pacing maneuvers and CARTO. J Cardiovasc Electrophysiol 2006; 17:1242–1245.
69. Tse HF, Reek S, Timmermans C, et al. Pulmonary vein isolation using transvenous catheter cryoablation for treatment of atrial fibrillation without risk of pulmonary vein stenosis. J Am Coll Cardiol 2003; 42:752–758.
70. Sarabanda AV, Bunch TJ, Johnson SB, et al. Efficacy and safety of circumferential pulmonary vein isolation using a novel cryothermal balloon ablation system. J Am Coll Cardiol 2005; 46:1902–1912.
71. Natale A, Pisano E, Shewchik J, et al. First human experience with pulmonary vein isolation using a through-the-balloon circumferential ultrasound ablation system for recurrent atrial fibrillation. Circulation 2000; 102:1879–1882.
72. Schmidt B, Metzner A, Chun KR, et al. Feasibility of circumferential pulmonary vein isolation using a novel endoscopic ablation system. Circ Arrhythm Electrophysiol 2010; 3:481–488.
73. Barrett CD, Natale A. Toward balloon-based technologies: All that glitters is not gold. J Cardiovasc Electrophysiol 2008; 19:952–954.
74. Ahsan SY, Flett AS, Lambiase PD, Segal OR. First report of phrenic nerve injury during pulmonary vein isolation using the ablation frontiers pulmonary vein ablation catheter. J Interv Card Electrophysiol 2010; 29:187–190.
75. Lee JC, Steven D, Roberts-Thomson KC, Raymond JM, Stevenson WG, Tedrow UB. Atrial tachycardias adjacent to the phrenic nerve: Recognition, potential problems, and solutions. Heart Rhythm 2009; 6:1186–1191.

76. Nakahara S, Ramirez RJ, Buch E, et al. Intrapericardial balloon placement for prevention of collateral injury during catheter ablation of the left atrium in a porcine model. Heart Rhythm 2010; 7:81–87.

77. Di Biase L, Burkhardt JD, Pelargonio G, et al. Prevention of phrenic nerve injury during epicardial ablation: Comparison of methods for separating the phrenic nerve from the epicardial surface. Heart Rhythm 2009; 6:957–961.

78. Gillinov AM, Pettersson G, Rice TW. Esophageal injury during radiofrequency ablation for atrial fibrillation. J Thorac Cardiovasc Surg 2001; 122:1239–1240.

79. Doll N, Borger MA, Fabricius A, et al. Esophageal perforation during left atrial radiofrequency ablation: Is the risk too high? J Thorac Cardiovasc Surg 2003; 125:836–842.

80. Pappone C, Oral H, Santinelli V, et al. Atrio-esophageal fistula as a complication of percutaneous transcatheter ablation of atrial fibrillation. Circulation 2004; 109:2724–2726.

81. Scanavacca MI, Avila AD, Parga J, Sosa E. Left atrial–esophageal fistula following radiofrequency catheter ablation of atrial fibrillation. J Cardiovasc Electrophysiol 2004; 15:960–962.

82. Cummings JE, Schweikert RA, Saliba WI, et al. Brief communication: Atrial–esophageal fistulas after radiofrequency ablation. Ann Intern Med 2006; 144:572–574.

83. Gilcrease GW, Stein JB. A delayed case of fatal atrioesophageal fistula following radiofrequency ablation for atrial fibrillation. J Cardiovasc Electrophysiol 2010; 21:708–711.

84. Ghia KK, Chugh A, Good E, et al. A nationwide survey on the prevalence of atrioesophageal fistula after left atrial radiofrequency catheter ablation. J Interv Card Electrophysiol 2009; 24:33–36.

85. Cummings JE, Schweikert RA, Saliba WI, et al. Assessment of temperature, proximity, and course of the esophagus during radiofrequency ablation within the left atrium. Circulation 2005; 112:459–464.

86. Lemola K, Sneider M, Desjardins B, et al. Computed tomographic analysis of the anatomy of the left atrium and the esophagus: Implications for left atrial catheter ablation. Circulation 2004; 110:3655–3660.

87. Ren JF, Lin D, Marchlinski FE, Callans DJ, Patel V. Esophageal imaging and strategies for avoiding injury during left atrial ablation for atrial fibrillation. Heart Rhythm 2006; 3:1156–1161.

88. Han J, Good E, Morady F, Oral H. Images in cardiovascular medicine. Esophageal migration during left atrial catheter ablation for atrial fibrillation. Circulation 2004; 110:e528.

89. Sause A, Tutdibi O, Pomsel K, et al. Limiting esophageal temperature in radiofrequency ablation of the left atrial tachyarrhythmias results in low incidence of thermal esophageal lesions. BMC Cardiovasc Disord 2010; 2652.

90. Zellerhoff S, Ullerich H, Lenze F, et al. Damage to the esophagus after atrial fibrillation ablation: Just the tip of the iceberg? High prevalence of mediastinal changes diagnosed by endosonography. Circ Arrhythm Electrophysiol 2010; 3:155–159.

91. Di Biase L, Dodig M, Saliba W, et al. Capsule endoscopy in examination of esophagus for lesions after radiofrequency catheter ablation: A potential tool to select patients with increased risk of complications. J Cardiovasc Electrophysiol 2010; 21:839–844.

92. Shah D, Dumonceau JM, Burri H, et al. Acute pyloric spasm and gastric hypomotility: An extracardiac adverse effect of percutaneous radiofrequency ablation for atrial fibrillation. J Am Coll Cardiol 2005; 46:327–330.

93. Abhishek F, Heist EK, Barrett C, et al. Effectiveness of a strategy to reduce major vascular complications from catheter ablation of atrial fibrillation. J Interv Card Electrophysiol 2011; 30:211–215.

94. Olsen DM, Rodriguez JA, Vranic M, Ramaiah V, Ravi R, Diethrich EB. A prospective study of ultrasound scan-guided thrombin injection of femoral pseudoaneurysm: A trend toward minimal medication. J Vasc Surg 2002; 36:779–782.

95. Sackett WR, Taylor SM, Coffey CB, et al. Ultrasound-guided thrombin injection of iatrogenic femoral pseudoaneurysms: A prospective analysis. Am Surg 2000; 66:937–940.

96. Ohlow MA, Secknus MA, von Korn H, et al. Incidence and outcome of femoral vascular complications among 18,165 patients undergoing cardiac catheterisation. Int J Cardiol 2009; 135:66–71.

97. Wittkampf FH, van Oosterhout MF, Loh P, et al. Where to draw the mitral isthmus line in catheter ablation of atrial fibrillation: Histological analysis. Eur Heart J 2005; 26:689–695.

98. Takahashi Y, Jais P, Hocini M, et al. Acute occlusion of the left circumflex coronary artery during mitral isthmus linear ablation. J Cardiovasc Electrophysiol 2005; 16:1104–1107.

99. Hinkle DA, Raizen DM, McGarvey ML, Liu GT. Cerebral air embolism complicating cardiac ablation procedures. Neurology 2001; 56:792–794.

100. Lesh MD, Coggins DL, Ports TA. Coronary air embolism complicating transseptal radiofrequency ablation of left free-wall accessory pathways. Pacing Clin Electrophysiol 1992; 15:1105–1108.

101. Le BH, Black JN, Huang SK. Transient ST-segment elevation during transseptal catheterization for atrial fibrillation ablation. Tex Heart Inst J 2010; 37:717–721.

102. Mofrad P, Choucair W, Hulme P, Moore H. Case report: Cerebral air embolization in the electrophysiology laboratory during transseptal catheterization: Curative treatment of acute left hemiparesis with prompt hyperbaric oxygen therapy. J Interv Card Electrophysiol 2006; 16:105–109.

103. Wu RC, Brinker JA, Yuh DD, Berger RD, Calkins HG. Circular mapping catheter entrapment in the mitral valve apparatus: A previously unrecognized complication of focal atrial fibrillation ablation. J Cardiovasc Electrophysiol 2002; 13:819–821.

104. Lakkireddy D, Nagarajan D, Di Biase L, et al. Radio frequency ablation (RFA) of atrial fibrillation in patients with mitral or aortic mechanical prosthetic valves—A feasibility, safety and efficacy study. Heart Rhythm 2011; 8:975–980.

105. Mountantonakis S, Frankel D, Hutchinson M, et al. Feasibility of catheter ablation of mitral annular flutter in patients with prior mitral valve surgery. Heart Rhythm 2011; 8:809–814.

106. Mansour M, Mela T, Ruskin J, Keane D. Successful release of entrapped circumferential mapping catheters in patients undergoing pulmonary vein isolation for atrial fibrillation. Heart Rhythm 2004; 1:558–561.

107. Je HG, Kim JW, Jung SH, Lee JW. Minimally invasive surgical release of entrapped mapping catheter in the mitral valve. Circ J 2008; 72:1378–1380.

108. Monney P, Pascale P, Fromer M, Pruvot E. Catheter entrapment in a pulmonary vein: A unique complication of pulmonary vein isolation. Chest 2010; 138:422–425.

109. Raviele A, Themistoclakis S, Rossillo A, Bonso A. Iatrogenic postatrial fibrillation ablation left atrial tachycardia/flutter: How to prevent and treat it? J Cardiovasc Electrophysiol 2005; 16:298–301.

110. Mesas C, Pappone C, Lang CCE, et al. Left atrial tachycardia after circumferential pulmonary vein ablation for atrial fibrillation: Electroanatomic characterization and treatment. J Am Coll Cardiol 2004; 44:1071–1079.

111. Chugh A, Oral H, Lemola K, et al. Prevalence, mechanisms, and clinical significance of macroreentrant atrial tachycardia during and following left atrial ablation for atrial fibrillation. Heart Rhythm 2005; 2:464–473.

112. Gerstenfeld EP, Callans DJ, Dixit S, et al. Mechanisms of organized left atrial tachycardias occurring after pulmonary vein isolation. Circulation 2004; 110:1351–1357.

113. Ouyang F, Antz M, Ernst S, et al. Recurrent pulmonary vein conduction as the dominant factor for recurrent atrial tachyarrhythmias after complete circular isolation of pulmonary veins: Lessons from double lasso technique. Circulation 2005; 111:127–135.

114. Deisenhofer I, Estner H, Zrenner B, et al. Left atrial tachycardia after circumferential pulmonary vein ablation for atrial fibrillation: Incidence, electrophysiological characteristics, and results of radiofrequency ablation. Europace 2006; 8:573–582.

115. Pappone C, Manguso F, Vicedomini G, et al. Prevention of iatrogenic atrial tachycardia after ablation of atrial fibrillation: A prospective randomized study comparing circumferential pulmonary vein ablation with a modified approach. Circulation 2004; 110:3036–3042.

116. Shah D, Sunthorn H, Burri H, et al. Narrow, slow-conducting isthmus dependent left atrial reentry developing after ablation for atrial fibrillation: ECG characterization and elimination by focal RF ablation. J Cardiovasc Electrophysiol 2006; 17:508–515.

117. Jais P, Hocini M, Hsu LF, et al. Technique and results of linear ablation at the mitral isthmus. Circulation 2004; 110:2996–3002.

118. Kanagaratnam L, Tomassoni G, Schweikert R, et al. Empirical pulmonary vein isolation in patients with chronic atrial fibrillation using a three-dimensional nonfluoroscopic mapping system: Long-term follow-up. Pacing Clin Electrophysiol 2001; 24:1774–1779.

119. Oral H, Scharf C, Chugh A, et al. Catheter ablation of paroxysmal atrial fibrillation. Segmental pulmonary vein ostial ablation versus left atrial ablation. Circulation 2003; 108:2355–2360.

120. Villacastín J, Pérez-Castellano N, Moreno J, González R. Left atrial flutter after radiofrequency catheter ablation of focal atrial fibrillation. J Cardiovasc Electrophysiol 2003; 14:417–421.

121. Ernst S, Ouyang F, Löber F, Antz M, Kuck KH. Catheter-induced linear lesions in the left atrium in patients with atrial fibrillation: An electroanatomic study. J Am Coll Cardiol 2003; 42:1271–1282.

122. Oral H, Chugh A, Lemola K, et al. Noninducibility of atrial fibrillation and an end point of left atrial circumferential ablation for paroxysmal atrial fibrillation: A randomized study. Circulation 2004; 110:2797–2801.

123. Cummings JE, Nassir NF, Schweikert R, et al. Left atrial flutter following pulmonary vein antrum isolation with radiofrequency energy: Linear lesions or repeat isolation. J Cardiovasc Electrophysiol 2005; 16:293–297.

124. Hocini M, Sanders P, Jais P, et al. Prevalence of pulmonary vein disconnection after anatomical ablation for atrial fibrillation; consequences of wide atrial encircling of the pulmonary veins. Eur Heart J 2005; 26:696–704.

125. Daoud EG, Weiss R, Augostini R, et al. Proarrhythmia of circumferential left atrial lesions for management of atrial fibrillation. J Cardiovasc Electrophysiol 2006; 17: 157–165.

126. Chae S, Oral H, Good E, et al. Atrial tachycardia after circumferential pulmonary vein ablation of atrial fibrillation: Mechanistic insights, results of catheter ablation, and risk factors for recurrence. J Am Coll Cardiol 2007; 50:1781–1787.

127. Sawhney N, Anousheh R, Chen W, Feld G. Circumferential pulmonary vein ablation with additional linear ablation results in an increased incidence of left atrial flutter compared with segmental pulmonary vein isolation as an initial approach to ablation of paroxysmal atrial fibrillation. Circ Arrhythm Electrophysiol 2010; 3:243–248.

128. Rostock T, Drewitz I, Steven D, et al. Characterization, mapping, and catheter ablation of recurrent atrial tachycardias after stepwise ablation of long-lasting persistent atrial fibrillation. Circ Arrhythm Electrophysiol 2010; 3:160–169.

129. Chang SL, Tsao HM, Lin YJ, et al. Differentiating macroreentrant from focal atrial tachycardias occurred after circumferential pulmonary vein isolation. J Cardiovasc Electrophysiol 2011; 22:748–755.

130. Brooks A, Stiles M, Laborderie J, et al. Outcomes of long-standing persistent atrial fibrillation ablation: A systematic review. Heart Rhythm 2010; 7:835– 846.

131. Gerstenfeld EP, Marchlinski FE. Mapping and ablation of left atrial tachycardias occurring after atrial fibrillation ablation. Heart Rhythm 2007; 4:S65–S72.

132. Karch MR, Zrenner B, Deisenhofer I, et al. Freedom from atrial tachyarrhythmias after catheter ablation of atrial fibrillation: A randomized comparison between 2 current ablation strategies. Circulation 2005; 111:2875–2880.

133. Anousheh R, Sawhney N, Panutich M, Tate C, Chen WC, Feld G. Effect of mitral isthmus block on development of atrial tachycardia following ablation for atrial fibrillation. Pacing Clin Electrophysiol 2010; 33:460–468.

134. Perez FJ, Wood MA, Schubert CM. Effects of gap geometry on conduction through discontinuous radiofrequency lesions. Circulation 2006; 113:1723–1729.

135. Thomas SP, Wallace EM, Ross DL. The effect of a residual isthmus of surviving tissue on conduction after linear ablation in atrial myocardium. J Interv Card Electrophysiol 2000; 4:273–281.

136. Lim TW, Koay CH, McCall R, See V, Ross DL, Thomas S. Atrial arrhythmias after single-ring isolation of the posterior left atrium and pulmonary veins for atrial fibrillation: Mechanisms and management. Circ Arrhythm Electrophysiol 2008; 1:120–126.

137. Chugh A, Oral H, Good E, et al. Catheter ablation of atypical atrial flutter and atrial tachycardia within the coronary sinus after left atrial ablation for atrial fibrillation. J Am Coll Cardiol 2005; 46:83–91.

138. Nademanee K, McKenzie J, Kosar E, et al. A new approach for catheter ablation of atrial fibrillation: Mapping of electrophysiologic substrate. J Am Coll Cardiol 2004; 43:2044–2053.

139. Gerstenfeld EP, Dixit S, Bala R, et al. Surface electrocardiogram characteristics of atrial tachycardias occurring after pulmonary vein isolation. Heart Rhythm 2007; 4:1136–1143.

140. Yamane T, Shah DC, Peng JT, et al. Morphological characteristics of P waves during selective pulmonary vein pacing. J Am Coll Cardiol 2001; 38:1505–1510.

141. Rajawat YS, Gerstenfeld EP, Patel VV, Dixit S, Callans DJ, Marchlinski FE. ECG criteria for localizing the pulmonary vein origin of spontaneous atrial premature complexes: Validation using intracardiac recordings. Pacing Clin Electrophysiol 2004; 27:182–188.

142. Chugh A, Latchamsetty R, Oral H, et al. Characteristics of cavotricuspid isthmus-dependent atrial flutter after left atrial ablation of atrial fibrillation. Circulation 2006; 113:609–615.

143. Jaïs P, Matsuo S, Knecht S, et al. A deductive mapping strategy for atrial tachycardia following atrial fibrillation ablation: Importance of localized reentry. J Cardiovasc Electrophysiol 2009; 20:480–491.

144. Patel AM, d'Avila A, Neuzil P, et al. Atrial tachycardia after ablation of persistent atrial fibrillation: Identification of the critical isthmus with a combination of multielectrode activation mapping and targeted entrainment mapping. Circ Arrhythm Electrophysiol 2008; 1:14–22.

145. Hall B, Jeevanantham V, Simon R, Filippone J, Vorobiof G, Daubert J. Variation in left atrial transmural wall thickness at sites commonly targeted for ablation of atrial fibrillation. J Interv Card Electrophysiol 2006; 17:127–132.
146. Becker AE. Left atrial isthmus: Anatomic aspects relevant for linear catheter ablation procedures in humans. J Cardiovasc Electrophysiol 2004; 15:809–812.
147. Tzeis S, Luik A, Jilek C, et al. The modified anterior line: An alternative linear lesion in perimitral flutter. J Cardiovasc Electrophysiol 2010; 21:665–670.
148. Merino JL. Slow conduction and flutter following atrial fibrillation ablation: Proarrhythmia or unmasking effect of radiofrequency application? J Cardiovasc Electrophysiol 2006; 17:516–519.
149. Jeevanantham V, Ntim W, Navaneethan SD, et al. Meta-analysis of the effect of radiofrequency catheter ablation on left atrial size, volumes and function in patients with atrial fibrillation. Am J Cardiol 2010; 105:1317–1326.
150. Reant P, Lafitte S, Jais P, et al. Reverse remodeling of the left cardiac chambers after catheter ablation after 1 year in a series of patients with isolated atrial fibrillation. Circulation 2005; 112:2896–2903.
151. Verma A, Kilicaslan F, Adams JR, et al. Extensive ablation during pulmonary vein antrum isolation has no adverse impact on left atrial function: An echocardiography and cine computed tomography analysis. J Cardiovasc Electrophysiol 2006; 17:741–746.
152. Nori D, Raff G, Gupta V, et al. Cardiac magnetic resonance imaging assessment of regional and global left atrial function before and after catheter ablation for atrial fibrillation. J Interv Card Electrophysiol 2009; 26:109–117.
153. Rodrigues AC, Scanavacca MI, Caldas MA, et al. Left atrial function after ablation for paroxysmal atrial fibrillation. Am J Cardiol 2009; 103:395–398.
154. Wilton S, Fundytus A, Ghali W, et al. Meta-analysis of the effectiveness and safety of catheter ablation of atrial fibrillation in patients with versus without left ventricular systolic dysfunction. Am J Cardiol 2010; 106:1284–1291.
155. Rosenthal LS, Beck TJ, Williams J, et al. Acute radiation dermatitis following radiofrequency catheter ablation of atrioventricular nodal reentrant tachycardia. Pacing Clin Electrophysiol 1997; 20:1834–1839.
156. Nahass GT. Fluoroscopy and the skin: Implications for radiofrequency catheter ablation. Am J Cardiol 1995; 76:174–176.
157. Lakkireddy D, Nadzam G, Verma A, et al. Impact of a comprehensive safety program on radiation exposure during catheter ablation of atrial fibrillation: A prospective study. J Interv Card Electrophysiol 2009; 24:105–112.
158. Efstathopoulos EP, Katritsis DG, Kottou S, et al. Patient and staff radiation dosimetry during cardiac electrophysiology studies and catheter ablation procedures: A comprehensive analysis. Europace 2006; 8:443–448.
159. Mahesh M. Fluoroscopy: Patient radiation exposure issues. Radiographics 2001; 21:1033–1045.
160. Kovoor P, Ricciardello M, Collins L, Uther JB, Ross DL. Risk to patients from radiation associated with radiofrequency ablation for supraventricular tachycardia. Circulation 1998; 98:1534–1540.
161. Perisinakis K, Damilakis J, Theocharopoulos N, Manios E, Vardas P, Gourtsoyiannis N. Accurate assessment of patient effective radiation dose and associated detriment risk from radiofrequency catheter ablation procedures. Circulation 2001; 104:58–62.
162. Chun KR, Wissner E, Koektuerk B, et al. Remote-controlled magnetic pulmonary vein isolation using a new irrigated-tip catheter in patients with atrial fibrillation. Circ Arrhythm Electrophysiol 2010; 3:458–464.

163. Arya A, Zaker-Shahrak R, Sommer P, et al. Catheter ablation of atrial fibrillation using remote magnetic catheter navigation: A case-control study. Europace 2011; 13:45–50.

164. Scaglione M, Biasco L, Caponi D, et al. Visualization of multiple catheters with electroanatomical mapping reduces X-ray exposure during atrial fibrillation ablation. Europace 2011; 13:955–962.

165. Bertaglia E, Bella PD, Tondo C, et al. Image integration increases efficacy of paroxysmal atrial fibrillation catheter ablation: Results from the CartoMerge Italian Registry. Europace 2009; 11:1004–1010.

166. Dragusin O, Weerasooriya R, Jaïs P, et al. Evaluation of a radiation protection cabin for invasive electrophysiological procedures. Eur Heart J 2007; 28:183–189.

167. Ross AM, Segal J, Borenstein D, Jenkins E, Cho S. Prevalence of spinal disc disease among interventional cardiologists. Am J Cardiol 1997; 79:68–70.

168. Goldstein JA, Balter S, Cowley M, Hodgson J, Klein LW. Occupational hazards of interventional cardiologists: Prevalence of orthopedic health problems in contemporary practice. Catheter Cardiovasc Interv 2004; 63:407–411.

CHAPTER 8

Short- and long-term efficacy of catheter ablation procedures for atrial fibrillation

Hugh Calkins[1], Emanuele Bertaglia[2], Antonio Berruezo[3], Aldo Bonso[4], Jonathan M. Kalman[5], Moussa Mansour[6], Atul Verma[7]

[1]Cardiology and Electrophysiology Department, The Johns Hopkins Hospital, Baltimore, MD, USA
[2]Cardiology Department, ULSS 13 Mirano, Mirano, Italy
[3]Cardiology Department, Clinic Hospital, Barcelona, Spain
[4]Cardiovascular Department, Dell'Angelo Hospital, Venice-Mestre, Italy
[5]Cardiology Department, Royal Melbourne and Western Hospitals, Melbourne, Australia
[6]Cardiac Arrhythmia Department, Massachusetts General Hospital, Boston, MA, USA
[7]Cardiology Department, Southlake Regional Health Center, Toronto, ON, Canada

Introduction

Since the last iteration of the Venice Chart Guidelines in 2007 [1], more data have become available describing the acute and long-term efficacies of catheter ablation for AF. In order to define the success rates of any given procedure, there must be a consistent approach to the technique, a well-accepted method of follow-up, and a strict definition of success. Earlier studies of AF ablation efficacy were limited by their heterogeneity in all of the above-mentioned criteria. Fortunately, over the last few years, guidelines have better characterized the definition of success and the minimum monitoring that must be performed postablation to detect AF recurrence. Data from multicenter trials have been published and several meta-analyses have pooled smaller studies to obtain aggregate success rates. These data provide a better understanding of the acute and long-term efficacy of AF ablation.

Definition of success

The Heart Rhythm Society Consensus Statement on ablation of AF published in 2007 helped provide much needed consistency in the way AF ablation

Atrial Fibrillation Ablation, 2011 Update: The State of the Art based on the VeniceChart International Consensus Document, First Edition. Edited by Andrea Natale and Antonio Raviele.
© 2011 John Wiley & Sons, Ltd. Published 2011 by John Wiley & Sons, Ltd.

studies were reported [2]. While there continues to be a variety of different techniques available for ablation, wide-antral isolation of the PVs has become the accepted "cornerstone" of any ablation procedure in clinical studies. For most studies in patients with paroxysmal AF, PVI is considered a sufficient endpoint for ablation. Additional substrate modification may be performed, such as linear ablation and/or targeting of CFE, but this has largely been reserved for patients with more persistent AF. The technologies used for performing ablation have proliferated (including irrigated-tip, balloon, and multipolar catheters as well as remote navigation systems), but the lesion sets and electrical endpoints have remained fairly consistent. The methods and intensity of patient monitoring continue to differ in studies, although most have conformed to the Consensus Statement recommendations that follow-up postablation should be a minimum of 12 months with ECGs and 24-hour Holter monitors at least every 3 months. The use of more meticulous methods for detecting AF (such as transtelephonic monitoring, external or implantable loop recorders) are likely to detect more AF, although there is some debate regarding the incidence of asymptomatic recurrence in previously highly symptomatic patients [3–6]. Regardless, most clinical trials have incorporated these more intensive monitoring techniques into their methodology. Finally, the definition of success has become more standardized. For the most part, early recurrences occurring within the first 3 months after the procedure are discounted as being due to inflammatory changes, part of the so-called blanking period. Recurrences after 3 months have been defined as episodes of AF lasting >30 seconds for reporting purposes, although the relevance of such short episodes of AF is not known. Success rates are also increasingly specifying the number of patients on and off AAD therapy postablation.

Acute efficacy of AF ablation

Acute recurrences of AF are not uncommon within the first 2–3 months postablation. Studies suggest that the incidence of early AF recurrence ranges from 35% to 50% [7–9]. These studies also show that most patients who go on to have late recurrence have usually had recurrence within the first 3 months, with early recurrence being one of the strongest predictors of late recurrence. However, as many as 50% of patients who have early recurrences will not continue to have AF in the longer term [7,8]. Hypothesized mechanisms for early recurrences include transient postablation atrial inflammation and/or incomplete healing of the lesion sets. Thus, most studies employ a blanking period during which early recurrences of AF or AFL are ignored. While most studies use a 3-month blanking, as suggested by the consensus document, other data have suggested that 2 months may be long enough given that early recurrences beyond that will predict later recurrence [10]. Many studies have also used temporary AA therapy during the blanking period to prevent early recurrences. The recently published 5A trial supports this early use of antiarrhythmics by demonstrating a reduction in early intervention and hospitalization while improving patient QoL [11].

Mid- to long-term efficacy of AF ablation

In patients with paroxysmal AF and minimal SHD, consistent success rates for catheter ablation can be achieved. In these patients, the success rate at 1-year off AADs is 60–75% after one procedure and 65–90% after two procedures. A number of recent systematic reviews have been published comparing the efficacy of catheter ablation of AF to AAD therapy [12–17]. In all of these reviews, the patient populations were predominantly, but not exclusively, paroxysmal (over 75%). Furthermore, the technique used in these studies was a wide-antral PVI technique with little to no adjuvant ablation performed. The results of all of these reviews showed superiority of RFA over AAD therapy with a success rate of 75.7–77% over 12 months when only randomized trials were included [15,16] and 71% when randomized trials were combined with prospective cohort studies [12] (Table 8.1). In many of these studies, a single repeat ablation procedure was required in 10–25% of patients. The data suggest that performing a second ablation procedure increases the chance of off-drug success by an additional 5–15% [18]. Whether more than two procedures provide benefit is not well known.

Since the last iteration of the Venice Chart Guidelines, a number of prospective, randomized studies on the longer term outcome of AF ablation have been published. In a single-center study, Pappone et al. reported an 86% single-procedure and 93% two-procedure freedom from atrial arrhythmia at 1 year compared with only 35% freedom in the AAD arm [19]. In a randomized study by Oral et al., 146 patients with permanent AF were randomized to circumferential ablation of the PVs or to electrical cardioversion with amiodarone for 3 months [20]. An intention-to-treat analysis revealed that 74% of the ablation-group patients and 58% of the controls were in sinus rhythm after 1 year ($p = .05$). In the CACAF multicenter, prospective study, patients in the ablation group had a significantly lower incidence of arrhythmic recurrence compared with those in the AA group (44% vs. 91%, $p < .001$) [21]. More recently, Jaïs et al. showed an 89% success rate at 1 year with catheter ablation (mean 1.8 ± 0.8 procedures) compared with 23% success for AADs ($p < .001, n = 112$) [22].

Table 8.1 Odds ratios and 95% confidence intervals of meta-analyses of success of catheter ablation of AF versus AAD therapy.

Study	Odds ratio	95% Confidence interval
Noheria et al. [15]	3.73	[2.47–5.63]
Nair et al. [14]	2.86	[1.75–4.76]
Piccini et al. [16]	15.78	[10.07–24.73]
Terasawa et al. [17]	3.46	[1.97–6.09]

In the STOP AF trial, which utilized cryoablation balloon technology for PVI, 245 patients were enrolled and the ablation group had a 69.9% success rate at 1 year (after one or more procedures) compared with only 7.3% success rate with AADs [23]. Finally, in a large, multicenter, randomized trial with RFA and an intensive postablation monitoring regimen, Wilber et al. published a 66% single-procedure success rate at 1 year compared with only 16% with AADs ($n = 167$) [24]. In an early pilot study, comparing first-line catheter ablation to AADs, Wazni et al. published that in 70 patients over 12 months, fewer symptomatic recurrences occurred in the ablation group (13% vs. 63%, $p < .001$) compared with AADs [25]. The full-sized RAAFT study will likely be published sometime this year. The very large CABANA study will also be comparing AF ablation to drug therapy in a higher risk cohort of 3000 patients enrolled across many centers worldwide, and while the trial is underway, results will not be available for a few years. A similar study will also be carried out exclusively in Europe called EAST, but this trial has yet to start enrollment at the time of writing this document.

Very long-term efficacy of AF ablation

Data on very long-term outcomes from AF ablation, beyond 1 year, are more limited and largely restricted to single-center experiences. A few studies have shown that outcome of AF ablation beyond 1 year is preserved. Weerasooriya et al. described one high-volume center's experience over 5 years of follow-up in both paroxysmal (63%) and persistent AF patients, showing that the majority of recurrences occur within 6 months of the ablation procedure. Success rates at 1, 2, and 5 years were 87%, 81%, and 63%, respectively, with a median of two procedures per patient [26]. Ouyang et al. reported similar results with a success rate of 79.5% in paroxysmal patients over 4.6 years of follow-up with only a 2.4% progression rate to chronic AF [27]. Medi et al. also showed that most recurrences occur within the first 6–12 months postablation and that success on drugs at 1 year is 87% and is still 80% at 4 years [28]. Another study showed that the occurrence of very late recurrence beyond 1 year was 1.7% [29], while Hunter et al. found a late recurrence risk of 3 per 100 patient years beyond 3 years of follow-up [30]. Risk factors for very late recurrence appear to be nonparoxysmal AF, valvular heart disease, cardiomyopathy, and advanced age [26].

However, other studies have published less optimistic results. Wokhlu et al. suggested that the risk of recurrence increased in absolute terms by 12% in paroxysmal patients and 20% in persistent patients from year 1 to year 2.5 [31]. Bertaglia et al. published that the actuarial atrial arrhythmia recurrence rate was 13.0% at 2 years, 21.8% at 3 years, 35.0% at 4 years, 46.8% at 5 years, and 54.6% at 6 years [32]. However, in both of these studies, the initial success rates were substantially lower than those reported in the previous section. Perhaps a difference in ablation technique is resulting in a higher late recurrence rate. Furthermore, although recurrences may be common, performing an additional procedure may still provide very long-term success. Sawhney et al., for example, showed that late recurrences after the first ablation were common, with an 86% success rate after 1 year, 79% after 2 years, and 56% after 5 years [33]. However, when additional ablation procedure(s) were performed on these patients, the success rate was still 81% off AADs at 63 ± 5 months of follow-up.

Efficacy in nonparoxysmal AF

In general, the success rate of AF ablation is lower in patients with persistent or long-standing persistent AF compared with paroxysmal AF. Many studies show success rates of 40–70% in nonparoxysmal AF and many have suggested the need for further adjuvant substrate modification in addition to PVI [34]. In a recently published meta-analysis of ablation in persistent AF, the pooled, single-procedure, drug-free success rate was only 44% in 211 patients who underwent wide-antral PVI alone [35]. With repeat procedures and concomitant drug therapy, the success rates increase to 59% and 77%, respectively. Addition of further adjuvant ablation may improve success rates. The drug-free, one-procedure success rate of PVI plus linear ablation ranges from 48% to 57% [35], which is better than the outcome data for PVI alone in persistent AF. As for PVI plus additional ablation of CFE, the result may also be better than that of PVI alone. When the results of the three available randomized studies are pooled (total 220 patients), the one-procedure success rate for PVI was 38% versus 51% for PVI plus CFE ablation and the two-procedure success rate was 72% and 77%, respectively [36–38]. However, further study is required to determine the optimal technique for ablating persistent AF, and this will be assessed in the ongoing STAR AF 2 trial.

Mechanisms of AF ablation failure

Studies have shown that the mechanism for longer term recurrence is linked to the recovery of electrical conduction between the PVs and the LA both in patients with paroxysmal and nonparoxysmal AF [39]. Recurrence, particularly AFL, may also be related to incomplete scars created by the initial ablation [40]. Thus, if ablation lesions, particularly linear lesions, are to be performed, it is critical to achieve complete block across these lines. Reisolation of the PVs is quite often effective in treating recurrent AF or AFL [41]. However, performance of additional ablation may be required, such as linear ablation or ablation of CFE, particularly in nonparoxysmal AF [42]. The mechanism of very late recurrences beyond 1 year may also involve development of non-PV triggers, either outside of the PV antra in the LA, or even within the CS and RA [29,43]. This process may be due to an evolving substrate as patients get older and as the AF becomes more chronic.

A number of clinical factors predict late failure of AF ablation. In particular, left atrial scarring may be the strongest predictor of procedural failure [44].

Evolving imaging techniques, particularly MRI, may help in identifying left atrial scar, thus risk stratifying patients prior to ablation so that the procedure can be performed only on those patients with the highest chance of success [45]. Other risk factors include significant left atrial enlargement, advanced age, nonparoxysmal AF, and SHD, such as cardiomyopathy or valvular heart disease [26,31,46,47]. Diabetes, hypertension, and sleep apnea syndrome have also been reported as risk factors for late recurrence, although not as consistently [8,31,48,49].

Conclusion

In summary, AF ablation appears to be an effective therapy over both the shorter and longer terms. Improvements are being made as to the uniformity of the ablation technique, definition of success, and rigor of follow-up. Additional multicenter, randomized data are still required and a number of large-scale trials are underway. Over the next 3–5 years, much more data will be available to more exactly define the success rates from this procedure. In particular, more prospective, multicenter data are required on very long-term outcomes beyond 1 year to assess the robustness of the procedure. AF ablation definitely appears to be superior to conventional drug therapy in controlling AF, but whether this translates into reduced morbidity and mortality remains to be seen and will be the subject of future trials.

References

1. Natale A, Raviele A, Arentz T, et al. Venice Chart international consensus document on atrial fibrillation ablation. J Cardiovasc Electrophysiol 2007; 18:560–580.
2. Calkins H, Brugada J, Packer DL, et al. HRS/EHRA/ECAS expert Consensus Statement on catheter and surgical ablation of atrial fibrillation: Recommendations for personnel, policy, procedures and follow-up. A report of the Heart Rhythm Society (HRS) Task Force on catheter and surgical ablation of atrial fibrillation. Heart Rhythm 2007; 4:816–861.
3. Oral H, Veerareddy S, Good E, et al. Prevalence of asymptomatic recurrences of atrial fibrillation after successful radiofrequency catheter ablation. J Cardiovasc Electrophysiol 2004; 15:920–924.
4. Hindricks G, Piorkowski C, Tanner H, et al. Perception of atrial fibrillation before and after radiofrequency catheter ablation: Relevance of asymptomatic arrhythmia recurrence. Circulation 2005; 112:307–313.
5. Steven D, Rostock T, Lutomsky B, et al. What is the real atrial fibrillation burden after catheter ablation of atrial fibrillation? A prospective rhythm analysis in pacemaker patients with continuous atrial monitoring. Eur Heart J 2008; 29:1037–1042.
6. Senatore G, Stabile G, Bertaglia E, et al. Role of transtelephonic electrocardiographic monitoring in detecting short-term arrhythmia recurrences after radiofrequency ablation in patients with atrial fibrillation. J Am Coll Cardiol 2005; 45:873–876.
7. Oral H, Knight BP, Ozaydin M, et al. Clinical significance of early recurrences of atrial fibrillation after pulmonary vein isolation. J Am Coll Cardiol 2002; 40:100–104.

8. Lee SH, Tai CT, Hsieh MH, et al. Predictors of early and late recurrence of atrial fibrillation after catheter ablation of paroxysmal atrial fibrillation. J Interv Card Electrophysiol 2004; 10:221–226.
9. Bertaglia E, Stabile G, Senatore G, et al. Predictive value of early atrial tachyarrhythmias recurrence after circumferential anatomical pulmonary vein ablation. Pacing Clin Electrophysiol 2005; 28:366–371.
10. Themistoclakis S, Schweikert RA, Saliba WI, et al. Clinical predictors and relationship between early and late atrial tachyarrhythmias after pulmonary vein antrum isolation. Heart Rhythm 2008; 5:679–685.
11. Roux JF, Zado E, Callans DJ, et al. Antiarrhythmics After Ablation of Atrial Fibrillation (5A Study). Circulation 2009; 120:1036–1040.
12. Calkins H, Reynolds MR, Spector P, et al. Treatment of atrial fibrillation with antiarrhythmic drugs or radiofrequency ablation: Two systematic literature reviews and meta-analyses. Circ Arrhythm Electrophysiol 2009; 2:349–361.
13. Gjesdal K, Vist GE, Bugge E, et al. Curative ablation for atrial fibrillation: A systematic review. Scand Cardiovasc J 2008; 42:3–8.
14. Nair GM, Nery PB, Diwakaramenon S, Healey JS, Connolly SJ, Morillo CA. A systematic review of randomized trials comparing radiofrequency ablation with antiarrhythmic medications in patients with atrial fibrillation. J Cardiovasc Electrophysiol 2009; 20:138–144.
15. Noheria A, Kumar A, Wylie JV, Jr., Josephson ME. Catheter ablation vs. antiarrhythmic drug therapy for atrial fibrillation: A systematic review. Arch Intern Med 2008; 168:581–586.
16. Piccini JP, Lopes RD, Kong MH, Hasselblad V, Jackson K, Al-Khatib SM. Pulmonary vein isolation for the maintenance of sinus rhythm in patients with atrial fibrillation: A meta-analysis of randomized, controlled trials. Circ Arrhythm Electrophysiol 2009; 2:626–633.
17. Terasawa T, Balk EM, Chung M, et al. Systematic review: Comparative effectiveness of radiofrequency catheter ablation for atrial fibrillation. Ann Intern Med 2009; 151:191–202.
18. Verma A, Natale A. Should atrial fibrillation ablation be considered first-line therapy for some patients? Why atrial fibrillation ablation should be considered first-line therapy for some patients. Circulation 2005; 112:1214–1222; discussion 1231.
19. Pappone C, Augello G, Sala S, et al. A randomized trial of circumferential pulmonary vein ablation versus antiarrhythmic drug therapy in paroxysmal atrial fibrillation: The APAF Study. J Am Coll Cardiol 2006; 48:2340–2347.
20. Oral H, Pappone C, Chugh A, et al. Circumferential pulmonary-vein ablation for chronic atrial fibrillation. N Engl J Med 2006; 354:934–941.
21. Stabile G, Bertaglia E, Senatore G, et al. Catheter ablation treatment in patients with drug-refractory atrial fibrillation: A prospective, multi-centre, randomized, controlled study (Catheter Ablation For The Cure Of Atrial Fibrillation Study). Eur Heart J 2006; 27: 216–221.
22. Jaïs P, Cauchemez B, Macle L, et al. Catheter ablation versus antiarrhythmic drugs for atrial fibrillation: The A4 study. Circulation 2008; 118:2498–2505.
23. Packer DL, Irwin JM, Champagne J, et al. Cryoballoon Ablation of Pulmonary Veins for Paroxysmal Atrial Fibrillation: First Results of the North American Arctic Front Stop-AF Clinical Trial *Presented at American College of Cardiology Meeting, Late Breaking Clinical Trials*, 2010.
24. Wilber DJ, Pappone C, Neuzil P, et al. Comparison of antiarrhythmic drug therapy and radiofrequency catheter ablation in patients with paroxysmal atrial fibrillation: A randomized controlled trial. JAMA 2010; 303:333–340.

25. Wazni OM, Marrouche NF, Martin DO, et al. Radiofrequency ablation vs antiarrhythmic drugs as first-line treatment of symptomatic atrial fibrillation: A randomized trial. JAMA 2005; 293:2634–2640.
26. Weerasooriya R, Khairy P, Litalien J, et al. Catheter ablation for atrial fibrillation: Are results maintained at 5 years of follow-up? J Am Coll Cardiol 2011; 57:160–166.
27. Ouyang F, Tilz R, Chun J, et al. Long-term results of catheter ablation in paroxysmal atrial fibrillation: Lessons from a 5-year follow-up. Circulation 2010; 122:2368–2377.
28. Medi C, Sparks PB, Morton JB, et al. Pulmonary vein antral isolation for paroxysmal atrial fibrillation: Results from long-term follow-up. J Cardiovasc Electrophysiol 2011; 22:137–141.
29. Miyazaki S, Kuwahara T, Kobori A, et al. Long-term clinical outcome of extensive pulmonary vein isolation-based catheter ablation therapy in patients with paroxysmal and persistent atrial fibrillation. Heart 2010; 97:668–673.
30. Hunter RJ, Berriman TJ, Diab I, et al. Long-term efficacy of catheter ablation for atrial fibrillation: Impact of additional targeting of fractionated electrograms. Heart 2010; 96:1372–1378.
31. Wokhlu A, Hodge DO, Monahan KH, et al. Long-term outcome of atrial fibrillation ablation: Impact and predictors of very late recurrence. J Cardiovasc Electrophysiol 2010; 21:1071–1078.
32. Bertaglia E, Tondo C, De Simone A, et al. Does catheter ablation cure atrial fibrillation? Single-procedure outcome of drug-refractory atrial fibrillation ablation: A 6-year multicentre experience. Europace 2010; 12:181–187.
33. Sawhney N, Anousheh R, Chen WC, Narayan S, Feld GK. Five-year outcomes after segmental pulmonary vein isolation for paroxysmal atrial fibrillation. Am J Cardiol 2009; 104:366–372.
34. Neumann T, Vogt J, Schumacher B, et al. Circumferential pulmonary vein isolation with the cryoballoon technique results from a prospective 3-center study. J Am Coll Cardiol 2008; 52:273–278.
35. Brooks AG, Stiles MK, Laborderie J, et al. Outcomes of long-standing persistent atrial fibrillation ablation: A systematic review. Heart Rhythm 2010; 7:835–846.
36. Verma A, Mantovan R, Macle L, et al. Substrate and trigger ablation for reduction of atrial fibrillation (STAR AF): A randomized, multicentre, international trial. Eur Heart J 2010; 31:1344–1356.
37. Elayi CS, Verma A, Di Biase L, et al. Ablation for longstanding permanent atrial fibrillation: Results from a randomized study comparing three different strategies. Heart Rhythm 2008; 5:1658–1664.
38. Oral H, Chugh A, Yoshida K, et al. A randomized assessment of the incremental role of ablation of complex fractionated atrial electrograms after antral pulmonary vein isolation for long-lasting persistent atrial fibrillation. J Am Coll Cardiol 2009; 53:782–789.
39. Verma A, Kilicaslan F, Pisano E, et al. Response of atrial fibrillation to pulmonary vein antrum isolation is directly related to resumption and delay of pulmonary vein conduction. Circulation 2005; 112:627–635.
40. Sawhney N, Anousheh R, Chen W, Feld GK. Circumferential pulmonary vein ablation with additional linear ablation results in an increased incidence of left atrial flutter compared with segmental pulmonary vein isolation as an initial approach to ablation of paroxysmal atrial fibrillation. Circ Arrhythm Electrophysiol 2010; 3:243–248.
41. Cummings JE, Schweikert R, Saliba W, et al. Left atrial flutter following pulmonary vein antrum isolation with radiofrequency energy: Linear lesions or repeat isolation. J Cardiovasc Electrophysiol 2005; 16:293–297.

42. Verma A. The techniques for catheter ablation of paroxysmal and persistent atrial fibrillation: A systematic review. Curr Opin Cardiol 2010.
43. Hsieh MH, Tai CT, Lee SH, et al. The different mechanisms between late and very late recurrences of atrial fibrillation in patients undergoing a repeated catheter ablation. J Cardiovasc Electrophysiol 2006; 17:231–235.
44. Verma A, Wazni OM, Marrouche NF, et al. Pre-existent left atrial scarring in patients undergoing pulmonary vein antrum isolation: An independent predictor of procedural failure. J Am Coll Cardiol 2005; 45:285–292.
45. Oakes RS, Badger TJ, Kholmovski EG, et al. Detection and quantification of left atrial structural remodeling with delayed-enhancement magnetic resonance imaging in patients with atrial fibrillation. Circulation 2009; 119:1758–1767.
46. Berruezo A, Tamborero D, Mont L, et al. Pre-procedural predictors of atrial fibrillation recurrence after circumferential pulmonary vein ablation. Eur Heart J 2007; 28:836–841.
47. Hof I, Chilukuri K, Arbab-Zadeh A, et al. Does left atrial volume and pulmonary venous anatomy predict the outcome of catheter ablation of atrial fibrillation? J Cardiovasc Electrophysiol 2009; 20:1005–1010.
48. Matiello M, Nadal M, Tamborero D, et al. Low efficacy of atrial fibrillation ablation in severe obstructive sleep apnoea patients. Europace 2010; 12:1084–1089.
49. Chilukuri K, Dalal D, Marine JE, et al. Predictive value of obstructive sleep apnoea assessed by the Berlin Questionnaire for outcomes after the catheter ablation of atrial fibrillation. Europace 2009; 11:896–901.

CHAPTER 9

Indications to atrial fibrillation ablation and cost-effectiveness

Eric N. Prystowsky[1], Josep Brugada[2], Samuel Lévy[3], Matthew Reynolds[4], Vincenzo Santinelli[5], Panos E. Vardas[6], Francesca Zuffada[5], Carlo Pappone[5]

[1]Clinical Electrophysiology Laboratory, St. Vincent Indianapolis Hospital, Indianapolis, IN, USA
[2]Cardiology Department, Thorax Institute, Clinic of Barcelona, Barcelona, Spain
[3]Cardiology Department, CHU Hôpital Nord, Marseille, France
[4]Beth Israel Deaconess Medical Center, Harvard Clinical Research Institute, Boston, MA, USA
[5]Arrhythmology Department, Villa Maria Cecilia Hospital, Cotignola, Italy
[6]Cardiology Department, Heraklion University Hospital, Heraklion, Greece

Indications to catheter ablation of AF

Several studies from experienced centers have demonstrated the efficacy of catheter ablation in patients with AF [1–12]. Therefore, catheter ablation of paroxysmal AF in symptomatic patients is an established indication in experienced centers after failure of antiarrhythmic drug therapy (Figure 9.1a), and LVF and LA size are important to define the class of recommendation according to guidelines for the management of patients with AF [13,14]. Class I, level of evidence A, is now recommended for patients with normal or mildly dilated LA and normal or mildly reduced LVF without severe pulmonary disease [14]. However, class IIa, level of evidence A, is recommended for patients with dilated LA or reduced LVF, and patients with paroxysmal AF and significant left atrial enlargement or significant LV dysfunction are class IIb [14]. Ablation of persistent AF is feasible [14] as second line treatment after failure of medical treatment (class IIa level of evidence A), but there is no real consensus since the procedure is more complex with a lower success rate (Figure 9.1b). For these reasons, catheter ablation of persistent AF requires a more accurate selection of patients and, particularly among patients with long-standing persistent AF, multiple interventions are frequently necessary to increase the success rate [8]. Thus, more data are needed to determine the

Atrial Fibrillation Ablation, 2011 Update: The State of the Art based on the VeniceChart International Consensus Document, First Edition. Edited by Andrea Natale and Antonio Raviele.
© 2011 John Wiley & Sons, Ltd. Published 2011 by John Wiley & Sons, Ltd.

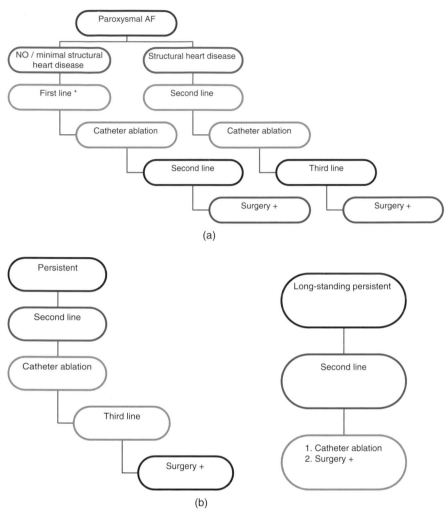

Figure 9.1 (a) Nonpharmacologic therapy of AF. Asterisk (∗) denotes selected patients (FA text), and plus symbol (+) denotes first line may be considered if the patient is undergoing cardiac surgery. (b) Nonpharmacologic therapy of AF.

most suitable candidates with long-standing AF for ablation (Figure 9.1b). A new class I first-line indication for catheter ablation of AF is proposed for selected patients with very symptomatic paroxysmal AF [11] (Figure 9.1a). This approach will require an accurate selection of candidates that includes patient preference for nonpharmacologic therapy, the absence (lone AF) or the presence of "minimal" SHD, relatively frequent AF, e.g., more than two episodes per month, and with operators that are very experienced. For these highly selected patients the ablative procedure may be performed at an earlier stage of the disease [9,11] to avoid or limit arrhythmia progression to more persistent forms [9], which is associated with lower success rate and with an increased need for repeat procedures.

Cost-effectiveness of catheter ablation

In industrialized countries, health care spending is an increasingly important economic and political issue. The discipline of cost-effectiveness analysis has developed over several decades as a tool for objectively assessing the value of new medical strategies, by simultaneously examining incremental health benefits in light of incremental costs. The core of cost-effectiveness analysis is the estimation of the difference in relative cost and efficacy (or effectiveness, that is real-world efficacy) of two compared therapeutic interventions. The underlying goal of cost-effectiveness research is to allow clinicians and policymakers to make more rational decisions regarding clinical care and resource allocation. Cost-effectiveness analysis is a type of economic evaluation that examines both the costs and outcomes (effects) of alternative intervention strategies comparing the cost of an intervention to its effectiveness as measured in health outcomes. The results are usually presented in ICER, which represents the additional cost of one unit of outcome gained by a new strategy, when compared with a competing strategy [15,16].

For a cost utility analysis, the outcomes of health care interventions are measured in units of health outcome that combine quality and quantity of life and can thus be compared between different interventions and health problems. The most well-known example of a measure of health utility is the quality-adjusted life year or QALY. Many favor the use of QALYs in cost-effectiveness studies because, at least in theory, they can be measured across a wide variety of health conditions. To calculate QALYs, one must measure utility weights, which reflect an individual's preference for a given health state on a scale ranging from 1.0 (perfect health) to 0 (death).

A person's (or population's average) utility may change over time and through the course of an illness. QALYs are calculated as utility multiplied by the length of time (in years) spent in the health state corresponding with that utility, summed over time.

Decision-makers are often faced with the challenges of resource allocation and at present, resources are scarce; therefore, they must be allocated judiciously. Unfortunately, limited data exist to help clinicians decide which of competing therapies in the management of the large and different patient population with AF is most appropriate. Although RFCA to treat AF is increasing rapidly worldwide, there are still limited data on cost-effectiveness of the procedure in comparison with AAD therapy, particularly in patients with persistent or long-standing persistent AF. Currently, several randomized trials have shown that in patients with paroxysmal AF, RFCA is superior to AADs in maintaining sinus rhythm mainly when offered as a second-line therapy. Recent data from randomized trials also suggest that RFCA as compared with AAD therapy may be associated with improved symptoms and QoL and lower hospitalization rates long term (4 years after randomization). Although cost-effectiveness models comparing catheter ablation to AADs have been developed, these models have been mostly applied to paroxysmal AF in which the ablation strategy is focused on electrical isolation of the PVs. Preliminary results of these studies suggest that RFCA is cost-effective in the short term (at 1 year), but there are no randomized data on long-term or lifetime benefits including improved QoL and reduction of the risk of stroke, heart failure, or death. Therefore, long-term cost-effectiveness analysis of RF ablation versus standard care therapy in AF is uncertain and not yet conclusive. Preliminary results refer to short- to medium-term time periods mainly in patients with baseline preserved QoL making ablation less attractive from a cost-effectiveness perspective despite elimination of AF. However, it is conceivable that ablation may be cost-effective also in the short- to medium-term in patients with paroxysmal AF and baseline poor QoL due to health illness other than AF (Figures 9.2 and 9.3). Prior study models of cost-effectiveness analysis, which mainly focused on patients with paroxysmal AF and without SHD, have assumed no benefit for ablation on the risk of stroke, heart failure, and death. Yet, if such a benefit will eventually be found in patients with paroxysmal, persistent or long-standing AF, the probability that RF ablation is "truly" cost-effective in the general AF population is much higher. Longer time horizons of analysis and increase of single-procedure efficacy worldwide would significantly improve the cost-effectiveness of RF ablation as compared with AAD therapy. Finally, another important but not well-defined question is to establish the appropriate timing for change in therapeutic strategy (AAD therapy vs. ablation) according to predefined failure of treatment strategy, and not just the time to first recurrence of AF.

This document will review available information on the cost-effectiveness of catheter ablation in the management of AF as well as areas of uncertainty requiring future development, research, and discussion. Additionally, cost-effectiveness analysis will be explored using appropriate disease simulation models in patients with paroxysmal, persistent, and long-standing AF in terms of arrhythmia recurrence, long-term maintenance of sinus rhythm, and morbidity including hospitalizations, adverse events, stroke, and QoL. Different studies have evaluated the total costs associated with AF ablation treatment. Weerasooriya et al. [17] in a single center study observed that the majority of the ablation costs were related to the ablation procedure, but with a further annual cost higher among AAD patients, resulting in AAD therapy total costs higher that continue to diverge over time. The authors have estimated that, over a 5-year period, the total cost of the ablation strategy reached was lower than the 5-year cost with a pharmacologic strategy (€6730 vs. €7194).

In 2006, Chan's US model [18] evaluated the cost-effectiveness of AF ablation compared with both rate control and AAD (amiodarone) treatment in different patient hypothetical cohorts (55-year-old and 65-year-old patient cohorts at moderate or low risk of stroke). The aim of the study was to determine what stroke risk reduction would be necessary for the procedure of

Cost-effectiveness evaluation

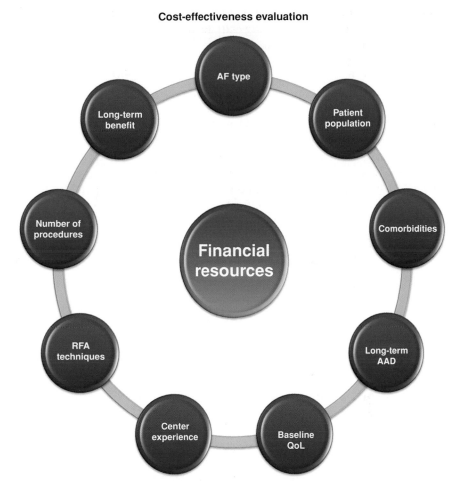

Figure 9.2 Cost-effectiveness analysis and financial resources in patients with AF. The figure shows that resources allocation should consider many variables including but not limited to AF type, the presence or absence of comorbidities, baseline QoL, and the center experience.

ablation to be cost-effective compared with rate control or AAD therapies. For the cohorts considered, Chan and colleagues calculated an ICER of ablation versus rate control of $28,700/QALY for 55-year-old patients at moderate risk of stroke, $51,800/QALY for 65-year-old moderate stroke risk patients, and an unfavorable $98,900/QALY for 65-year-old low stroke risk patients. These data are based on the fact that the authors have considered a range of reductions in stroke and mortality following conversion to NSR, which is assumed to be achieved by a higher percentage of ablation patients than by patients following any other treatment strategy: 78% of ablated patients were in NSR after 1 year compared with approximately 36% and 58% of rate control and amiodarone patients, respectively; therefore, patients in NSR have stroke risks

Cost-effective strategy of catheter ablation of AF

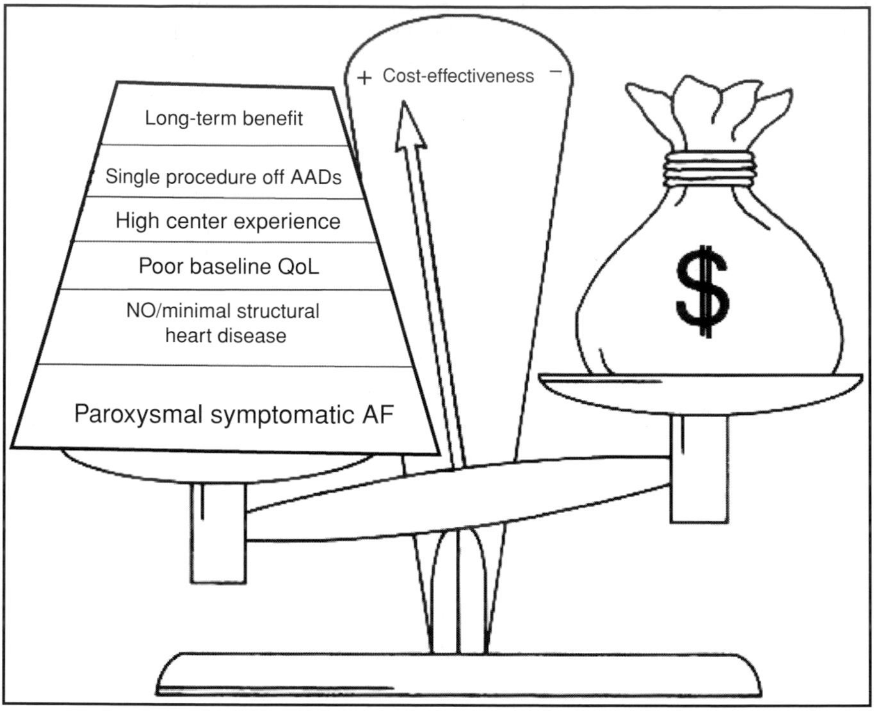

Figure 9.3 RFCA and cost-effectiveness analysis. The figure shows that RFA is cost-effective in patients with paroxysmal AF, no or minimal structural heart disease and poor baseline QoL, but long-term benefits and a single procedure are required.

ranging from 0.5% to 0.9% compared with 0.7% to 2.3% for patients in AF, and patients experiencing a stroke have a mortality percentage of 8.2–17.9%. The presumed reductions in stroke are hypothetical and need further study. Total calculated lifetime costs are higher for patients undergoing ablation, and ranged from $43,036 to $59,380 for ablation compared with $24,540 to $50,509 for rate control and $38,425 to $55,795 for amiodarone.

Khaykin et al. [19], comparing the costs of AF catheter ablation with the cost of rate control or AAD treatment, concluded that costs of ablation and AAD therapy would be equal after 3.2–8.4 years of follow-up, or with 3% discounting applied, after 4.5–10.8 years of follow-up.

Rodgers et al. [20–22] evaluated the cost-effectiveness of AF ablation from the UK health care system perspective. In their base-case scenario, the authors estimated lifetime costs of £26,027 for ablation and £15,367 for AAD treatment. The starting point was the assumption of procedure cost of £9810 and AAD costs of £186 in the first year, and then £32 per year thereafter. Annual treatment costs were assumed to be equal for both NSR and AF (£646 per year).

In 2009, an economic analysis of the RAAFT pilot study in Canada [21] compared the costs of AF ablation with AADs in the treatment of symptomatic paroxysmal AF. After the first year of follow-up, costs were $12,283 in the ablation arm and $6053 in the AAD arm with an important difference in the rate of hospitalizations in favor of AF ablation (9% vs. 54%). After 2 years costs for patients in the AA arm were $14,392 for AADs versus $15,303 for ablation. After this period of observation, AAD patients were allowed to undergo ablation. These 2-year AAD additional costs accurately represent the cost of a delayed ablation strategy. From the point of view of the US health care system, Reynolds et al. [23] assessed the cost-effectiveness of AF relying on data from literature and AF ablation costs and QoL outcomes. $15,000 was the estimated cost for AF ablation, with annual follow-up costs of $1300 in year 1 and $200 in later years if NSR was maintained. Like previous studies, over a 5-year time horizon, ablation was found to cost more than therapy with AADs (US$26,584 vs. US$19,898), and the authors noted that the initial higher costs of ablation were partly offset by lower long-term costs.

The potential cost-effectiveness of RFA for AF, relative to AAD therapy, is important because decision-making is also based on economic considerations. A cost-effectiveness study was conducted from the third party payer's perspective (INHS) to compare RFA and AAD therapy in patients with paroxysmal AF. A comparison was made of the 1-year follow-up data from the 198 patients of the APAF study (JACC 2006) [1] who were randomly assigned to catheter ablation (99 patients) or to new AAD therapy (99 patients) [24]. Efficacy and direct medical costs were quantified. Sensitivity analyses were conducted to account for the uncertainties as well as to identify how estimates could vary under different assumptions for CV events. Costs paid by the hospital to perform RFA were quantified and compared with the reimbursement provided by NHS. At the time of analyses (2009), 1 euro (€) corresponded to around US$1.41. In 1 year, RFA cost was on average €6923/patient, while AAD treatment was €6773/patient. RFA cost driver was the cost of the procedure (82.9% of total costs), while AAD cost driver was the cost of hospitalizations for cardiovascular reasons (48% of total costs). Using RFA generated an ICER of €239/patient AF-free and an ICER of €25/patient-month AF-free (€149/6.02 patient-months). Under different assumptions for CV events, RFA strategy appeared to be dominant (i.e., contemporarily more effective and less costly) in a best case hypothesis (up to €2000/patient saved in 1 year), or, in a worst case hypothesis, it could generate an ICER up to €800/patient AF-free and €85/patient-month AF-free.

If the real costs are reimbursed to the hospital, the ICER increases to €7000/patient AF-free and to €736/patient-month free from AF gained. In conclusion, it appears that RFA among patients with paroxysmal AF who have already failed AAD therapy is cost-effective in just 1-year follow-up. However, currently RFA is much more costly to the provider hospital than the reimbursement received from INHS. If to perform RFA a reimbursement congruent with real costs is provided, the offset of costs could be reached in a few years. Therefore, on the basis of the evidence presented above, it can be argued that a single catheter ablation procedure can be a cost-attractive alternative to pharmacotherapy over time by decreasing subsequent long-term health care expenses, despite the initial high procedural ablation cost. However, this argument is limited by the lack of robust long-term data pertaining to the efficacy of a single AF ablation procedure in long-term studies, particularly in patients with persistent or long-standing AF. The CABANA trial [25], a randomized controlled trial comparing AF ablation to rate control or AAD medication, began enrolling patients in August 2009. CABANA has been designed with a planned enrollment of 3000 AF patients who will be followed for a minimum of 2 years, and the trial will prospectively gather data on mortality, stroke, and other clinical outcomes in a broad AF patient population, addressing many of the limitations of the current clinical evidence base. CABANA will also collect data on health economic and QoL outcomes. Completion of CABANA is expected in 2015.

Other factors may affect the cost-effectiveness of AF ablation. Very late AF recurrences requiring multiple ablation procedures and associated health care expenditures requires further study. The underestimation of asymptomatic arrhythmia recurrence is another factor that modifies the cost-effectiveness. The cost of complications is important. In the worldwide survey, the complication rate was 6% with four early deaths, while in a recent study of 1101 consecutive patients the respective percentage was 3.9% [26]. Experience also matters, and higher volume centers tend to have fewer major complications and better long-term outcomes, both of which will be favorable to AF cost-effectiveness. One should also remember that amiodarone, the most frequently prescribed drug to maintain sinus rhythm in AF patients, has several side effects, some life-threatening, that occur over time. The costs to the health care system both in performing routine surveillance tests to identify amiodarone organ toxicity and to treat such events when they occur is not trivial, and such cost data need to be put into the overall analysis.

Further information to evaluate the cost-effectiveness of the ablation procedure is related to the heterogeneity of the patient population with AF as well as to the limited generalizability of data among patient subgroups included in clinical trials and treated in high-volume centers. These patients likely do not constitute a representative sample of the general patient population with AF, while the advanced level of health care provided in the specialized centers may improve efficacy and safety but may also increase the related treatment cost. Thus, any attempt at extrapolation of the calculated cost and cost- effectiveness measures is prone to biases. Furthermore, considerable differences in unit prices and resource utilization among different centers and, importantly, among different countries impair a cost calculation that could be representative of all European countries or other parts of the world. The assumptions used to construct cost-effectiveness models have a noteworthy impact on determining which patients might be the most cost-effective candidates for ablation. If one assumes that the major health benefits for ablation over alternative treatments are reductions in stroke and mortality risk, as in the Chan et al. [18] model, then ablation will appear most cost-effective in patients with at least a moderately elevated risk of stroke. However, if QALY gains following ablation are driven primarily by improvements in symptoms and QoL associated solely with maintenance of sinus rhythm, then the optimal ablation candidate from a cost-effectiveness standpoint is somewhat different. Under this set of assumptions, cost-effectiveness is most likely in patients with lower baseline QoL scores (i.e., patients highly symptomatic from their AF) who lack major comorbid conditions, since impaired QoL due to other health problems might be less likely to respond to catheter ablation.

References

1. Pappone C, Augello G, Sala S, et al. A randomized trial of circumferential pulmonary vein ablation versus antiarrhythmic drug therapy in paroxysmal atrial fibrillation: The APAF study. J Am Coll Cardiol 2006; 48:2340–2347.
2. Jaïs P, Cauchemez B, Macle L, et al. Catheter ablation versus antiarrhythmic drugs for atrial fibrillation: The A4 study. Circulation 2008; 118:2498–2505.
3. Wilber DJ, Pappone C, Neuzil P, et al. ThermoCool AF Trial Investigators. Comparison of antiarrhythmic drug therapy and radiofrequency catheter ablation in patients with paroxysmal atrial fibrillation: A randomized controlled trial. JAMA 2010; 303:333–340.
4. Ouyang F, Tilz R, Chun J, et al. Long-term results of catheter ablation in paroxysmal atrial fibrillation. Lessons from a 5-year follow-up. Circulation 2010; 122:2368–2377.
5. Hsu LF, Jaïs P, Sanders P, et al. Catheter ablation for atrial fibrillation in congestive heart failure. N Engl J Med 2004; 351:2373–2383.
6. Reynolds MR, Walczak J, White SA, Cohen DJ, Wilber DJ. Improvements in symptoms and quality of life in patients with paroxysmal atrial fibrillation treated with radiofrequency catheter ablation versus antiarrhythmic drugs. Circ Cardiovasc Qual Outcomes 2010; 3:615–623.
7. Sawhney N, Anousheh R, Chen WC, Narayan S, Feld GK. Five-year outcomes after segmental pulmonary vein isolation for paroxysmal atrial fibrillation. Am J Cardiol 2009; 104:366–372.
8. Bhargava M, Di Biase L, Mohanty P, et al. Impact of type of atrial fibrillation and repeat catheter ablation on long-term freedom from atrial fibrillation: Results from a multicenter study. Heart Rhythm 2009; 6:1403–1412.
9. Pappone C, Radinovic A, Manguso F, et al. Atrial fibrillation progression and management: A 5-year prospective follow-up study. Heart Rhythm 2008; 5:1501–1507.
10. Oral H, Pappone C, Chugh A, et al. Circumferential pulmonary-vein ablation for chronic atrial fibrillation. N Engl J Med 2006; 354:934–941.
11. Wazni OM, Marrouche NF, Martin DO, et al. Radiofrequency ablation vs antiarrhythmic drugs as first line treatment of symptomatic atrial fibrillation: A randomized trial. JAMA 2005; 293:2634–2640.
12. Stabile G, Bertaglia E, Senatore G, et al. Catheter ablation treatment in patients with drug refractory atrial fibrillation: A prospective, multicentre, randomized, controlled study (Catheter Ablation for the Cure of Atrial Fibrillation Study). Eur Heart J 2006; 27:216–221.
13. Fuster V, Rydén LE, Cannom DS, et al. ACC/AHA/ESC 2006 guidelines for the management of patients with atrial fibrillation: Executive summary: A report of the American

College of Cardiology/American Heart Association Task Force on Practice Guidelines and the European Society of Cardiology Committee for Practice Guidelines. J Am Coll Cardiol 2006; 48:854–906.

14. Wann LS, Curtis AB, January CT, et al.; ACCF/AHA/HRS. ACCF/AHA/HRS focused update on the management of patients with atrial fibrillation (Updating the 2006 Guideline): A report of the American College of Cardiology Foundation/American Heart Association Task Force on Practice Guidelines. J Am Coll Cardiol 2011; 57:223–242.

15. Goodacre S, McCabe C. An introduction to economic evaluation. Emerg Med J 2002; 19:198–201.

16. Cohen DJ, Reynolds MR. Interpreting the results of cost-effectiveness studies. J Am Coll Cardiol 2008; 52:2119–2126.

17. Weerasooriya R, Jaïs P, Le Heuzey JY, et al. Cost analysis of catheter ablation for paroxysmal atrial fibrillation. Pacing Clin Electrophysiol 2003; 26:292–294.

18. Chan PS, Vijan S, Morady F, Oral H. Cost-effectiveness of radiofrequency catheter ablation for atrial fibrillation. J Am Coll Cardiol 2006; 47:2513–2520.

19. Khaykin Y, Morillo CA, Skanes AC, McCracken A, Humphries K, Kerr CR. Cost comparison of catheter ablation and medical therapy in atrial fibrillation. J Cardiovasc Electrophysiol 2007; 18:907–913.

20. Rodgers M, McKenna C, Palmer S, et al. Curative catheter ablation in atrial fibrillation and typical atrial flutter: Systematic review and economic evaluation. Health Technol Assess 2008; 12:iii–iv. xi–xiii, 1–198.

21. Khaykin Y, Wang X, Natale A, et al. Cost comparison of ablation versus antiarrhythmic drugs as first-line therapy for atrial fibrillation: An economic evaluation of the RAAFT pilot study. J Cardiovasc Electrophysiol 2009; 20:7–12.

22. McKenna C, Palmer S, Rodgers M, et al. Cost-effectiveness of radiofrequency catheter ablation for the treatment of atrial fibrillation in the United Kingdom. Heart 2009; 95:542–549.

23. Reynolds MR, Zimetbaum P, Josephson ME, Ellis E, Danilov T, Cohen DJ. Cost-effectiveness of radiofrequency catheter ablation compared with antiarrhythmic drug therapy for paroxysmal atrial fibrillation. Circ Arrhythm Electrophysiol 2009; 2:362–369.

24. Santinelli V, Vicedomini G, Zuffada F, et al. Catheter ablation versus antiarrhythmic drug therapy in paroxysmal AF: A cost-effectiveness analysis. Abstract presented at the American College of Cardiology New Orleans, April 2–5, 2011.

25. Clinical Trials.gov. Identifier NCT00911508: Ablation Versus Anti-Arrhythmic (AA) Drug Therapy for AF-Pivotal Trial (CABANA). Bethesda, MD: National Library of Medicine. http://clinicaltrialsgov/ct2/show/NCT00911508. Accessed on July 2010.

26. Cappato R, Calkins H, Chen SA, et al. Worldwide survey on the methods, efficacy, and safety of catheter ablation for human atrial fibrillation. Circulation 2005; 111:1100–1105.

CHAPTER 10

Clinical trials on atrial fibrillation/ future perspectives

A. John Camm[1], Carina Blomström-Lundqvist[2], Paul Dorian[3], Stefan H. Hohnloser[4], Carlos A. Morillo[5], Pasquale Santangeli[6], Isabelle C. van Gelder[7], Erik Wissner[8], Paulus Kirchhof[9]

[1]Cardiac and Vascular Sciences, St. George's Hospital Medical School, London, UK
[2]Cardiology Department, University Hospital in Uppsala, Uppsala, Sweden
[3]Cardiology Department, St. Michael's Hospital, Toronto, ON, Canada
[4]Electrophysiology Department, J.W. Goethe University, Frankfurt, Germany
[5]Arrhythmia & Pacing Department, Hamilton General Hospital, Hamilton, ON, Canada
[6]Texas Cardiac Arrhythmia Institute, St. David's Medical Center, Austin, TX, USA
[7]Cardiology Department, University Medical Center Groningen, Groningen, The Netherlands
[8]Cardiology Department, Asklepios Klinik St. Georg, Hamburg, Germany
[9]Chair in Cardiovascular Medicine, School of Clinical & Experimental Medicine, University of Birmingham, Birmingham, UK

AF ablation was introduced into clinical practice as an experimental technique that can be used compassionately to alleviate symptoms in patients with extreme suffering, most often patients with paroxysmal AF [1]. Later, standardization of ablation techniques, technical improvements, and the wider-spread use of this technique have firmly established AF ablation as an important component of rhythm-control management in AF patients [2–5]. In this chapter, we will first discuss the evidence that supports the current role of AF ablation in the management of AF, and then take a look at planned and ongoing trials that may shape the future role of AF ablation.

Catheter ablation compared with AADs as technique to maintain sinus rhythm

Catheter ablation should be considered when AAD therapy has failed to control the patient's symptoms or proved intolerable in a patient with symptomatic AF [6]. In this context, catheter ablation has gained a class Ia

Atrial Fibrillation Ablation, 2011 Update: The State of the Art based on the VeniceChart International Consensus Document, First Edition. Edited by Andrea Natale and Antonio Raviele.
© 2011 John Wiley & Sons, Ltd. Published 2011 by John Wiley & Sons, Ltd.

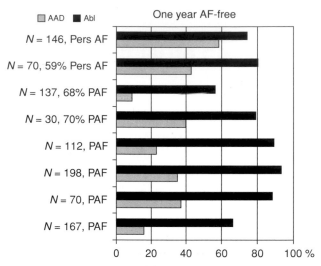

Figure 10.1 The eight randomized, controlled studies (from top of figure; (9)ₓ(14) (7–8, 10–13)) comparing AF ablation and AAD treatment in patients with symptomatic AF. Figures to the right denote efficacy rates. Abl denotes ablation, Pers denotes persistent AF, and *N* denotes number.

recommendation in latest US guidelines, while in European guidelines is considered class IIa indication. There are eight randomized controlled trials, in which left atrial catheter ablation have been compared with AAD medication with regard to maintenance of sinus rhythm in patients with symptomatic AF (Figure 10.1). In four of these studies, >95% of patients had paroxysmal AF [7–10]. Three others included both types of AF [11–13] and one study included only patients with persistent AF [14].

The inclusion criteria in seven of these studies was failure to respond to AAD treatment, which usually included 1–2 drugs [7–14]. There was thus only one study, in which ablation was compared with AADs as first-line treatment in patients with recurrent AF. All of the studies showed that AF ablation was superior to AADs in preventing recurrent AF at 9 months to 1 year of follow-up. PVI, with or without additional linear lesions, prevented recurrence of AF in 56–93% of the cases. The corresponding figures for patients allocated to the AAD group were 9–58%. The efficacy rates varied between 39% and 64% for paroxysmal and between 16% and 37% for persistent AF, all in favor of ablation (Table 10.1). Most studies achieved these results without continued AAD therapy beyond the blinding period of up to 3 months after the ablation. Some studies reported their results after only one ablation procedure, while others made the comparison after a period of monitoring during which the patient could be treated once or several times with ablation if needed (Table 10.1). The relatively large variation in treatment efficacy rates (16–64% units) can be attributed to differences in patient selection including types of AF, choice of drug strategy in the control group, treatment technologies, ablation

Table 10.1 Randomized, controlled studies comparing AF ablation using RF energy and AAD treatment of symptomatic AF.

AF type (%), year of publication, reference	Ablation technique	Number of patients		Results • Sinus rhythm (% without symptomatic AF) • QoL vs. AAD • Symptom vs. AAD • Hospitalization vs. AAD		Efficacy Rate %	Follow-up time Procedures/patient % with AA drugs		
		Abl	AAD	Abl	AAD		Months	Abl N	AAD%
PAF 96%, 2005 [9]	PVI	33	37	87 QoL ☐ (6 months) Hospital ☐	37	50	12	1	12%
PAF, 2006 [8] #	Anatomical w/wo XLL	99	99	93 QoL ☐ Hospital ☐	35	58	12	1.1	0%
PAF, 2008 [7] #	PVI w/wo XLL	53	59	87	23	64	12	1.8	0%
PAF, 2010 [10] #	PVI w/wo XLL	106	61	66 QoL ☐ Symptoms ☐	16	50	9	1.1	7,5%

(Continued)

Table 10.1 (Continued)

AF type (%), year of publication, reference	Ablation technique	Number of patients		Results • Sinus rhythm (% without symptomatic AF) • QoL vs. AAD • Symptom vs. AAD • Hospitalization vs. AAD		Efficacy Rate %	Follow-up time Procedures/patient % with AA drugs		
		Abl	AAD	Abl	AAD		Months	Abl N	AAD%
PAF 70%, 2003 [12]	PVI w XLL	15	15	79 QoL□ Symptoms□	40	39	12	NA	NA
PAF 67%, 2006 [13] #	Anatomical w/wo XLL	68	69	56 Hospital ns	9	47	12	1	100%
Pers AF 59%, 2009 [11]	PVI w/wo XLL	35	35	80 QoL□ Hospital□	43	37	12	1	0%
Pers AF, 2006 [14] #	Anatomical w XLL	77	69	74 Symptoms□	58	16	12	1.3	0%

Notes:
# denotes studies with 42–77% cross-over rates in the AAD arm.
Abl denotes ablation arm.
□/□ denotes significantly increased/decreased.
w/wo denotes with/without.
N denotes number of procedures.
Ns denotes nonsignificant.
Pers denotes persistant AF.
Sympt denotes symptom.

experience, and criteria for treatment efficacy. A difference in patient selection between the studies is evident by the relatively large variation in response rates among patients allocated to AAD treatment (Figure 10.1).

It is also worth mentioning that a strict ITT analysis was used in the study that only included patients with persistent AF [14]. Because a high proportion (77%) of patients in the drug arm crossed over to the ablation arm, the efficacy rate seemed smaller as compared with the other studies, which used an on-treatment analysis. It should also be emphasized that since most of these randomized studies were conducted at high-volume centers with many years of experience of AF ablation, the reported efficacy rates may not reflect the results achieved in smaller ablation centers.

In some of these studies, PV isolation was combined with additional pre-determined electrically isolating lines between the PVs, the MV, or inside the CS to improve patient outcomes (Table 10.1). A disadvantage of this approach is an increased risk of left atrial macroreentry tachycardia, i.e., regular rapid rhythm disturbances around areas in the LA where the insulation is incomplete. Electrical isolation of all PVs is currently the standard method shown to be most effective against recurrences of paroxysmal AF [15].

In general, the exclusion criteria in these studies were patients with valvular disease or mechanical valve prostheses, previous open-heart surgery, age over 70–75 years, permanent AF, patients with impaired LVF or heart failure, left atrial diameter of >55–65 mm, pacemakers, or previous history of stroke. Therefore, it is difficult to determine whether the reported results of treatment are for the above patient groups.

QoL, symptoms, and hospitalization

All five randomized trials (Table 10.1) that analyzed the effects on QoL have shown significantly greater improvement in QoL for patients undergoing AF ablation than for those who only received AAD treatment. Most patients evaluated by the QoL questionnaire SF-36 reported greater improvement in general and/or physical function. All three studies that used symptom questionnaires could demonstrate that symptoms were also more favorably affected by ablation than by AADs. Moreover, the hospitalization rate was significantly lower in patients in the ablation group compared with the AAD group, as shown in three of the four studies that examined the number of readmissions to hospital (Table 10.1).

Even though the clinical indication for treatment of AF is to eliminate or reduce symptoms related to the arrhythmia, none of these eight studies used symptoms or QoL as the primary endpoint. Instead, measures of AF recurrences, most commonly a 30 seconds AF episode, were used as the primary endpoint. Brief episodes of AF, however, do not necessarily translate into reduced QoL or the need for a new ablation procedure. Recurrences of AF may after an ablation procedure be asymptomatic or improve to such an extent that another intervention is not desired. The use of recurrent arrhythmias or

AF burden as primary endpoints, thus seem more relevant in trials evaluating new ablation techniques.

Other limitations with the trials were that in several studies the technique of randomization was not given, the results were not blinded, power-calculation was missing, <90% of patients were followed, patient selection criteria and measures of variability were lacking, as were reports on missing patients and information on prospective recruitment of patients.

Meta-analyses of randomized trials comparing catheter ablation and AAD treatment

There are several meta-analysis based on randomized trial that compared AF ablation with AAD treatment [16–21]. All six analyses confirmed the superiority of AF ablation versus AADs to achieve freedom from AF, reduced symptoms and fewer hospitalizations, even when corrected for the great heterogeneity between the studies.

Effect on survival and TEs

No attempts were made to evaluate the effect on long-term survival and thromboembolic complications in these randomized controlled studies, as the number of patients included was too small and the follow-up time was too short. In a nonrandomized controlled study comparing AF ablation and preventive drug therapy, patients treated with ablation had lower mortality than those who received continued drug treatment during a follow-up of 900 days [22]. The mortality rate after ablation was 7.4% lower in patients with coronary artery disease and left ventricular dysfunction. After 3 years of follow-up, heart failure and strokes were less frequent (8% and 17%, respectively) and the proportion of recurrences was lower (22% and 63%) after treatment with ablation compared with drug therapy [22]. Since the study was not randomized, it is uncertain whether the patients in the ablation and drug group were comparable. A meta-analysis of the eight randomized trials including 930 patients could, however, not demonstrate any differences in mortality or thromboembolic morbidity between the catheter ablation and AAD groups [16]. Large randomized studies are required to reliably ascertain whether left atrial ablation reduce mortality and/or risk of TEs in AF.

Complications

Complications are generally more common during AAD treatment but seem less severe than those observed with catheter ablation [23]. Treatment with catheter ablation thus carries some risk for serious complications and its risk profile differs from that of continued pharmacotherapy.

Serious complications occur in 4–5% of patients treated by catheter ablation. The most serious complication following ablation in the posterior wall of the LA involves development of a fistula between the LA and the esophagus [16,24]. Other serious complications include cardiac tamponade (1%), vascular complications (1–2%), thromboembolism/stroke (1–1.5%), PN paralysis (1–5%), and PV stenosis (1–2%). Factors associated with an increased complication risk is age over 75 years, female gender, heart failure, and staff with limited experience of surgery [16].

Economic aspects

Available randomized studies comparing drugs and ablation provide limited information on long-term effects and have in general rhythm as the primary endpoint. Therefore, the scientific evidence is insufficient for drawing conclusions about the cost-effectiveness of the method, since its long-term effects are uncertain.

Finally, a major limitation that partly explains the superiority of ablation versus AADs in these trials, is the fact that in all studies except one [9], patients had already failed several AADs when entering into the study. Therefore, it is not surprising that patients randomized to continuous AAD treatment, albeit with a new drug, had higher failure rates in maintaining sinus rhythm and higher rate of cross-over rates than the patients in the ablation group [14].

Further studies that compare the two treatment alternatives at an earlier stage of the AF diseases are, therefore, needed before conclusions can be made for the implementation of the results into clinical practice.

Perspectives onto measuring QoL in AF trials

QoL is important to measure as an outcome in AF, given that the primary purpose of AF ablation procedures is to improve general well-being and QoL. Until morbidity and mortality are shown to be reduced in controlled trials of AF ablation, the benefits on QoL will continue to be the dominant benefits expected from this procedure.

Prior studies of AF have generally not focused on measurements of QoL, and rather focused on recurrences of AF either clinically or electrocardiographically. Because some episodes of AF maybe minimally symptomatic and patients may have ongoing symptoms despite "success" in eliminating AF, an independent evaluation of AF related symptoms and associated QoL is necessary to gain a full understanding of the potential benefits of the procedure on QoL and well-being.

Most prior studies which did measure QoL used generic instruments such as the SF-36 or the euroqol (EQ-5D), which are "generic" instruments that measure QoL aspects related to general well-being, mobility, activities, social and physical functioning, but not necessarily specifically related to AF. In most studies of AF, it is preferable to measure QoL using "disease specific" questionnaires, which can more directly assess symptoms related to AF itself or its treatment.

Examples of AF specific measurements of QoL include the symptom check list [25], the University of Toronto AFSS, the new and recently validated AFEQT scale [26], all of which are patient self-administered, as well as the physician administered Severity of AF scale (CCS-SAF) [27]; the EHRA score is similar in concept and measurement to the CCS-SAF class [4,28].

To best understand the effect of ablation on QoL in AF, it is useful to have a baseline measure of QoL, preferably not immediately prior to the ablation procedure (since the expectation of an upcoming surgical procedure may alter QoL in and of itself), as well as QoL measurements in follow-up, e.g., at 3, 6, or 12 months after the procedure. Importantly, QoL will be affected not only by the procedure but also by ongoing other therapies, and may be differently affected in patients requiring more than one ablation procedure, or those with complications. Finally, it must be recognized that that in any nonblinded procedure such as AF, there will be treatment expectation effects that may be separate and independent of the rhythm outcomes of ablation. Thus, even in randomized controlled studies of RFA, some of the QoL outcomes may be related to nonspecific effects of treatment expectation from the ablation procedure, rather than direct effects of the ablation itself. An example of such "treatment expectancy" effects is the demonstration of a reduction in vasovagal syncope when pacemaker therapy was compared with no pacemaker therapy (VPSI study), an effect that disappeared when patients and caregivers were blinded to pacemaker therapy [29]. Most of the ongoing larger trials of AF ablation will use such disease-specific instruments to assess QoL.

Perspectives onto ongoing trials on catheter ablation of AF

Multiple ongoing randomized trials are further evaluating the benefit of catheter ablation over AAD therapy for rhythm control of AF in populations not included in published trials. In addition to the prevention of AF recurrence and improving symptoms and QoL, additional endpoints have also been considered important in recent years to evaluate the role of AF catheter ablation. These include reduction of hospitalization, stroke, and mortality, the safety of the procedure, as well as economic factors. A correct assessment of these endpoints has required the design of new clinical trials adequately powered to address these issues. Here, we provide an overview of the known trials that attempt to further our understanding of the clinical value of AF ablation. For simplicity, trials have been classified according to common endpoints of interest (Table 10.2).

Trials focused on mortality, hospitalizations, and stroke

CABANA
Designed as a randomized, multicenter, international, open label study, the CABANA trial [30] intends to test the hypothesis of whether left atrial catheter ablation for the treatment of AF is superior to pharmacological therapy in

Table 10.2 List of trials involving catheter ablation and AF as indicated in clinicaltrials.gov (n = 113, February 23, 2011), sorted by number of patients. Trials aiming at technical improvements have not been listed.

Study and STATUS	Main study question	Number of patient	Start	Duration	End follow-up	Primary outcome	Investigational intervention	QoL	LVF measured	Clinical trial accession number
Catheter ablation vs. AAD therapy for AF trial. RECRUITING	The CABANA trial is designed to test the hypothesis that the treatment strategy of left atrial catheter ablation for the purpose of eliminating AF will be superior to current state-of-the-art therapy with either rate-control or rhythm-control drugs for reducing total mortality in patients with untreated or incompletely treated AF.	3000	08/09	03/15	09/15	Total mortality.	Left atrial ablation compared with AAD therapy.	X	X	NCT 00911508
Early therapy of AF for STroke prevention trial (EAST) will start recruiting before publication of the document.	Can an early rhythm-control intervention improve hard outcomes compared with usual care in AF patients?	2810	6/10	2016		A composite of cardiovascular death, stroke, myocardial infarction, or decompensated heart failure.	Early rhythm-control therapy (catheter ablation and AADs directly after the diagnosis) added to usual care.			NCT 01288352

(Continued)

Table 10.2 (Continued)

Study and STATUS	Main study question	Number of patient	Start	Duration	End follow-up	Primary outcome	Investigational intervention	QoL	LVF measured	Clinical trial accession number
Catheter ablation vs. standard conventional treatment in patients with left ventricular dysfunction and AF. RECRUITING	In patients with heart failure, catheter ablation could improve cardiac function, symptoms, and QoL. It remains still unknown whether AF ablation is more effective than conventional treatment in terms of mortality and morbidity.	420	01/08	04/15		All-cause mortality or worsening heart failure requiring unplanned hospitalization.	RFA of AF.	X		NCT 00643188
First-line RFA vs. AADs for AF treatment: a multicenter randomized trial. RECRUITING	Study is to determine whether catheter-based PVI is superior to AADs as first-line therapy in patients with symptomatic paroxysmal recurrent AF not previously treated with therapeutic doses of AADs.	400	08/06	12/09		Time to first recurrence of AF. Ablation arm: severe (>70%) PV stenosis at 3- and 12-month follow-up. TE with residual sequelae, TIA, pericarditis, myocardial infarction, diaphragmatic paralysis, procedural complication requiring intervention and death. AAD arm: Torsade de Pointes, syncope, bradycardia	Procedure: PVI. Drug: control group receives AADs per ACC/AHA 2006 Guidelines for the management of patients with AF.	X	X	NCT 00392054

Study	N	Start	End	Purpose	Outcome	Intervention		NCT
					requiring pacemaker, other proarrhythmic events, any other significant adverse events leading to drug discontinuation. Bleeding complications associated with OAC therapy.			
AF after cardiac surgery—prospective, randomized study comparing conventional and miniaturized bypass systems. RECRUITING	330	07/10	12/13	The purpose of the study is to find out the difference in the incidence of AF when using the conventional (CECC) or mini bypass system (MECC).	Incidence of AF.	Procedure: miniaturized bypass system.		NCT 01160393
Medical AA treatment or RFA in paroxysmal AF: a randomized prospective multicentre study (MANTRA-PAF). RECRUITING	300	09/05	12/10	The present study is a prospective, randomized, multicenter study comparing medical AAD strategy with catheter-based RF strategy in patients with paroxysmal AF.	AF burden.	RFA vs. AAD therapy.		NCT 00133211
The effect of short-term amiodarone treatment after catheter ablation for AF. RECRUITING	250	01/09	02/12	To examine the overall effectiveness of short-time AAD treatment with amiodarone (to control heart rhythm)	Freedom from AF, AFL, or atrial tachycardia.	Catheter ablation with or without amiodarone treatment after ablation.	X	NCT 00826826

(Continued)

Table 10.2 (Continued)

Study and STATUS	Main study question	Number of patient	Start	Duration	End follow-up	Primary outcome	Investigational intervention	QoL	LVF measured	Clinical trial accession number
	to prevent short- and long-term AF following an ablation procedure for AF.									
AF management in CHF with ablation. RECRUITING	To compare the effect of best medical treatment of AF with primary catheter ablation by left linear PVI on LVEF in patients with a reduced ejection fraction of <35% requiring ICD/CRTD implantation and symptomatic AF.	216	01/08	07/11		LVEF as determined by TTE.	Early AF ablation vs. usual care in patients after defibrillator implantation.		X	NCT 00652522
The value of add-on arrhythmia surgery in patients with paroxysmal or persistent AF undergoing valvular or coronary bypass surgery. A randomized comparison on QoL, cost-effectiveness, morbidity, and rhythm outcome. COMPLETED	The hypothesis being studied is that add-on arrhythmia surgery in patients with AF undergoing valvular or coronary surgery improves QoL, is cost-effective, reduces perioperative and long-term morbidity associated with AF.	150	09/02	11/06	12/06	Percentage of patients free from AF, as apparent from 24-hour Holter registration, in addition to standard ECG. For the purpose of this primary endpoint, AF was defined as lasting longer than 10 seconds.	Procedure: PVI.	X		NCT 01019759

Trial / Status	Purpose	N	Start			Primary outcome	Comparison		NCT number
Randomized comparison of RFCA vs. AA therapy with amiodarone for maintaining sinus rhythm in patients with CAF. COMPLETED	The purpose of this study is to determine the long-term efficacy of RFCA in patients with CAF.	140	11/02	02/05		Freedom from AF and AFL in the absence of AAD therapy at 1 year.	RFCA compared with amiodarone therapy and cardioversion.	X	NCT 00272636
RFCA for CAF. COMPLETED	The purpose of this study is to determine the long-term efficacy of RFCA in patients with CAF.	140	10/02	02/05		Freedom from AF and AFL in the absence of AAD therapy at 1 year.	Catheter ablation vs. cardioversion and AAD therapy.	X	NCT 00272636
Study of Ablation Versus antiaRrhythmic Drugs in Persistent Atrial Fibrillation (SARA) RECRUITING	The purpose of this study is to compare the effectiveness and safety of atrial fibrillation ablation, in comparison to antiarrhythmic drug therapy in patients with refractory, persistent atrial fibrillation.	208	03/09	03/11	03/12	Freedom from atrial arrhythmias, lasting more than 24 hours or requiring cardioversion.	Atrial Fibrillation ablation (at least PV isolation) vs. Antiarrhythmic drugs	X	NCT 00863213
Randomized comparison of RFCA vs. AA therapy with amiodarone for maintaining sinus rhythm in patients with CAF. COMPLETED	The purpose of this study is to determine the long-term efficacy of RFCA in patients with CAF.	140	11/02	02/05		AF and AFL in the absence of AAD therapy at 1 year.	RFCA vs. amiodarone and cardioversion.	X	NCT 00272636

(Continued)

Table 10.2 (Continued)

Study and STATUS	Main study question	Number of patient	Start	Duration	End follow-up	Primary outcome	Investigational intervention	QoL	LVF measured	Clinical trial accession number
Randomized study comparing cardioversion vs. catheter ablation in patients with persistent AF. RECRUITING	The aim of this randomized study is to evaluate the efficacy of two different approaches for conversion of persistent AF, the noninvasive one (external electrical cardioversion) and the invasive one (catheter ablation).	130	08/05	06/09	12/09	Event-free survival after 6 months (i.e., freedom of atrial tachyarrhythmias—as evaluated in a 7-d Holter, stroke, PV stenosis—as evaluated in a CT-/MRT-scan 6 months after the initial procedure— and death).	Catheter ablation vs. external electric cardioversion.	X		NCT 00196209
Ablation vs. amiodarone for treatment of AF in patients with CHF and an implanted ICD/CRTD. RECRUITING	To determine if catheter-based AF ablation is superior to amiodarone treatment for symptomatic persistent/permanent AF in ICD/CRTD patients with an impaired LVF.	120	10/08	08/10	08/11	Time to recurrence of AF lasting longer than 15 seconds.	AF ablation RF catheter ablation of AF vs. amiodarone therapy in patients who received a defibrillator.	X	X	NCT 00729911
Clinical and economic consequences of left atrial bipolar RFA of persistent and permanent AF of cardiac surgery. TERMINATED	The study will examine if and to what extent the QoL and the use of medical care differs between patients with and without ablation.	100	09/05				QoL cost of care.	Intraoperative bipolar RFA of persistent and permanent AF compared with management without ablation.	X	X	NCT 00157807

Description	N				Primary outcome	Comparison			NCT
Sinus rhythm maintenance in patients with HCM and AF—randomized comparison of AA therapy vs. RFCA (SHAARC). RECRUITING	90	01/09	03/11	09/11	Freedom from AF and AFL (>1 minute) on or off AA medications.	RF catheter ablation vs. AADs.	X		NCT 00821353
Randomized controlled trial of PV antrum isolation vs. AVN ablation with biventricular pacing vs. PVI for treatment of AF in patients with congestive heart failure (PABA CHF). COMPLETED	81	11/02	11/06		Composite of EF, 6-minute walk distance, and MLWHF score.	PVI vs. AVN ablation in patients with heart failure and AF.			NCT 00599976
A randomized trial to assess catheter ablation vs. rate control in the management of persistent AF in chronic heart failure. RECRUITING	80	04/09	10/11	10/11	Peak oxygen consumption at cardiopulmonary exercise test [time frame: 12 months] [designated as safety issue: no].	Catheter ablation vs. rate-control therapy.	X	X	NCT 00878384

(Continued)

Table 10.2 (Continued)

Study and STATUS	Main study question	Number of patient	Start	Duration	End follow-up	Primary outcome	Investigational intervention	QoL	LVF measured	Clinical trial accession number
Catheter ablation vs. AAD therapy for AF—pilot trial. COMPLETED	CABANA is designed to test the hypothesis that the treatment strategy of percutaneous left atrial catheter ablation for the purpose of the elimination of AF is superior to current state-of-the-art therapy with either rate control or AADs for reducing total mortality (primary endpoint) and decreasing the composite endpoint of total mortality, disabling stroke, serious bleeding, and cardiac arrest (secondary endpoint) in patients with untreated or incompletely treated AF warranting therapy.	60	09/06	02/09	06/10	Percutaneous left atrial catheter ablation for the purpose of eliminating AF is superior to current state-of-the-art therapy with either rate or rhythm-control drugs for reducing total mortality in patients with untreated or undertreated AF.	Pharmacologic therapy rate and/or rhythm control Device: NAVI-STAR thermo-cool (left atrial catheter ablation).	X		NCT 00578617
PVI for rhythm control in patients with AF and left ventricular dysfunction RECRUITING	To compare heart function, symptoms, exercise capacity, and QoL in patients with CHF and AF before and after catheter ablation.	50	04/10	03/12	03/14	Improvement in LVESV by 15% or more from baseline at 6 months.	PVI, no control group.	X		NCT 01082601

terms of all-cause mortality. Secondary outcome parameters include rate of cardiovascular death, disabling stroke, serious bleeding, cardiovascular hospitalization, left atrial size, morphology and function, freedom of recurrent AF, as well as health economic parameters and QoL. The CABANA trial began enrolling patients in August 2009 and as of May 2011, over 200 patients have been enrolled. The target population comprises 3000 patients who are referred to participating centers for rhythm-control therapy of AF. The data of the pilot trial have been presented and demonstrated that enrollment is feasible. To some extent, there was a slant of disappointment because the actual rate of maintaining sinus rhythm in the patients enrolled into the pilot trial was lower than anticipated. By design, the CABANA trial will answer the questions whether catheter ablation improves mortality compared with AAD therapy, and will hence provide important information on the value of catheter ablation compared with AAD therapy beyond symptom and rhythm control. The hypothesis of the trial is based on observational data and suggests that catheter ablation can prevent relevant outcomes for AF such as stroke and death [28].

EAST

The EAST tests the hypothesis that an early, structured rhythm-control therapy can reduce morbidity and mortality in AF patients compared with usual care. The trial is jointly conducted by the German AFNET and the EHRA. Basis of the trial is the observation that AF-induced damage to the atria is often irreversible in patients with a long AF history [28,31], resulting in less effective rhythm-control therapy. Furthermore, the rate of AF-related complications is highest in the first year after diagnosis [32,33]. The trial will enroll patients with recent-onset AF (<12 months duration) at risk for cardiovascular events. Patients will be randomized to early rhythm-control therapy consisting of AADs or catheter ablation and supplementation of the therapy with the other therapeutic modality upon AF recurrence. This early rhythm-control therapy will be compared with usual care following the 2010 ESC guidelines on AF. The EAST investigators expect to enroll the first patient this summer. While CABANA compares two types of rhythm-control therapy (catheter ablation and AAD therapy), EAST compares a novel therapeutic strategy to usual care. This new therapeutic strategy, called "early and comprehensive rhythm-control therapy", applies catheter ablation and AADs at an early point in time when they are still likely to be effective. This early intervention is pursued with the hope that preventing AF recurrences can prevent severe outcomes associated with AF such as stroke and death.

The potential benefits of early rhythm-control therapy have recently been outlines in several review and opinion papers [34–37], and many arrhythmia specialists share the impression that an early initiation of rhythm-control therapy has potential benefits. However, this assumption, which has some biological plausibility, has never been put to test. EAST will address whether a structured, "comprehensive", early rhythm-control therapy can improve relevant outcomes in patients with AF in a large, controlled, randomized, multicenter trial.

Both CABANA and EAST are prospective, randomized, open-label, blinded outcome assessment (PROBE) trials. Industry-independent sponsors (DUKE and AFNET) and trial planning and initiation by investigators from academia are further structural similarities that render both trials credible. CABANA will give an answer to the burning questions whether catheter ablation can improve rhythm-control therapy to an extent that mortality can be reduced. EAST will answer the question whether adding rhythm-control therapy to current AF management can improve "hard outcomes" in AF patients. Both trials are thereby clearly supplementing each other. The coordinating investigators have agreed to plan combined analyses of the trial data sets once they become available, and it appears likely that combined analyses of the trial results will give further insights into the impact of treating AF on severe outcomes associated with the arrhythmia.

CASTLE-AF

This controlled, open, randomized trial studies whether catheter ablation can improve outcomes, mainly based on hospitalizations and QoL, in patients who receive a cardiac resynchronization device. These patients will be randomized to catheter ablation (including repeated ablations following a dedicated protocol) or usual care after device implantation. By design, this trial will enroll patients with advanced heart failure, similar to the outcomes of two smaller patient series that were enrolled in selected centers [38,39], and contrasts the interpretation of a large registry of CRT patients in whom AV nodal ablation appeared the most beneficial therapeutic option for AF in these patients [40]. CASTLE-AF is a multicenter trial that will provide valuable on the impact of catheter ablation for AF in the management of CRT recipients.

Trials testing the effectiveness of catheter ablation early in the treatment of AF

RAAFT-2

The first-line RAAFT-2 study is a randomized controlled trial comparing PV isolation versus AADs as a first-line therapy in patients with symptomatic recurrent paroxysmal AF not previously treated with therapeutic doses of AADs. The RAAFT-2 trial has been conceived after the promising results of the pilot RAAFT-1 trial, which randomized 70 patients with symptomatic AF (96% paroxysmal) to PV antrum isolation or AAD therapy as a first-line therapy. At the end of the 1-year follow-up, 63% of patients assigned to AAD therapy experienced at least one recurrence of symptomatic AF, as compared with 13% of those assigned to the PV antrum isolation treatment arm ($p <$ .001). Moreover, PV antrum isolation was associated with a significantly lower rate of hospitalization (9% vs. 54%, $p <$ .001) and better QoL [9]. As mentioned, the RAAFT-2 will enroll patients with recurrent paroxysmal AF lasting

>30 seconds (at least four episodes within the prior 6 months) without ev-
idence of left ventricular hypertrophy or dysfunction (i.e., left ventricular
ejection fraction <40%), significant left atrial enlargement (>5.5 cm), or contraindication to AA or antithrombotic drug therapy. The primary efficacy endpoint will be the time to first recurrence of AF. The results of the RAAFT-2 will
add further evidence toward the appropriateness of including PV isolation
among the evidence-based first-line therapies for symptomatic AF.

MANTRA-PAF

The Radiofrequency Ablation Versus Antiarrhythmic Drug Treatment in
Paroxysmal Atrial Fibrillation (MANTRA-PAF) is a randomized trial comparing PV isolation versus AAD therapy in patients with paroxysmal AF who are
considered as being candidates for AAD therapy. The primary efficacy endpoint is reduction of AF burden, while among important safety endpoints are
mortality, complications of treatment, QoL, and economic factors. The design
of the MANTRA-PAF is similar to that of the RAAFT-2, and shares with the
latter the same key exclusion criteria, namely, left ventricular dysfunction and
significantly enlarged left atria.

Trials of AF ablation in patients with heart failure

AATAC

The AATAC and an ICD/CRTD is a physician-initiated multicenter randomized trial comparing catheter ablation of AF versus amiodarone for symptomatic persistent/permanent AF in patients with ICD/CRTD and left ventricular dysfunction. To be eligible for enrollment in the AATAC, patients need
to have evidence of left ventricular dysfunction (i.e., left ventricular ejection
fraction ≤40%), a dual chamber ICD/CRTD, and symptomatic persistent or
CAF resistant to AAD therapy other than amiodarone. The primary efficacy
endpoint is the time to recurrence of AF lasting longer than 15 seconds, as assessed by cardiac device interrogation. Among secondary endpoints, there are
the distance walked in the 6-minute walk test, hospitalizations, and change in
left ventricular ejection fraction during the trial period. Preliminary results of
this trial, which have been recently presented in abstract form [41], suggest
a superiority of catheter ablation of AF over amiodarone to achieve freedom
from AF at follow-up.

AMICA

The AMICA trial will randomize patients with severe left ventricular dysfunction (i.e., ejection fraction ≤35%) and symptomatic persistent or long-standing
persistent AF undergoing ICD/CRTD implantation to catheter ablation of
AF or state-of-the-art optimal medical therapy. The primary endpoint of the
AMICA will be changes in left ventricular ejection fraction during the study
follow-up. This endpoint will be analyzed also in the AATAC trial and is of
relevant clinical importance. Indeed, if catheter ablation will be demonstrated

to improve the LVF, catheter ablation would be a reasonable attempt in patients with AF and values of left ventricular dysfunction close to the guideline suggested cutoff of 35% before the implantation of a prophylactic ICD/CRTD.

ARC-HF

The aim of the Catheter ARC-HF is to assess the optimal treatment of AF in patients with heart failure. At variance with the AATAC and AMICA trials, the ARC-HF will compare rhythm-control therapy with catheter ablation versus medical rate-control therapy. Basically, the design of the ARC-HF is similar to the large pharmacologic trial AF-CHF [42], which randomized a total of 1376 patients with a left ventricular ejection fraction of 35% or less, symptoms of CHF, and AF to either pharmacologic rhythm- or rate-control therapy. The AF-CHF trial showed that pharmacologic rhythm-control therapy does not reduce the risk of death, stroke, or worsening heart failure compared with a rate-control therapy [42]. Notably in the AF-CHF, the rhythm-control strategies adopted were not actually demonstrated to effectively maintain sinus rhythm. Disturbingly, the absolute difference in percentage of patients in sinus rhythm during follow-up in the AF-CHF trial was of only 40%, since sinus rhythm was not maintained in 100% of the patients in the rhythm-control group and was maintained in some of the patients in the rate-control group. Up to 58% of patients in the rhythm-control group had at least one recurrence of AF during follow-up. Moreover, the use of AADs in the rhythm-control arm is certainly questionable in terms of safety, and probably contributed to the lack of benefit in this group. With these premises, the ARC-HF trial is important as it tests a safe rhythm-control strategy, namely, catheter ablation, potentially eliminating the confounding contributions of low efficacy and high toxicity associated with AAD therapy at least in those patients who will remain free from AF recurrence off drugs. However, the major drawback of this trial is its inadequate power to address hard endpoints such as mortality and hospitalization. The primary endpoint tested will be changes in peak oxygen consumption at cardiopulmonary exercise test. Freedom from AF recurrence, changes in left ventricular ejection fraction and in exercise tolerance will be among the secondary endpoints analyzed.

Trials of AF ablation in patients with persistent and long-standing persistent AF

SARA

The SARA is evaluating the effectiveness and safety of catheter ablation of AF in comparison to AAD therapy in patients with symptomatic persistent AF. Overall, 208 patients with symptomatic persistent AF will be randomized to catheter ablation with PV isolation plus adjunctive strategies at the discretion of the enrolling hospitals versus state-of-the-art AAD therapy. Among key exclusion criteria, there is significant left atrial enlargement (i.e., left atrial diameter >5.0 cm) or left ventricular dysfunction (i.e., left ventricular ejection fraction <30%). The follow-up duration will be 1 year, with a primary efficacy endpoint of time from recurrent persistent AF. Recurrences of nonpersistent AF, total burden of AF, hospitalizations, and QoL will be included among the secondary endpoints. The results of the SARA will help clarifying whether catheter ablation should be considered as the optimal rhythm-control therapy in patients with persistent AF.

Radiofrequency catheter ablation for chronic AF

This multicenter randomized trial will compare catheter ablation of AF with amiodarone treatment and cardioversion in patients with CAF without significant left atrial enlargement (i.e., left atrial diameter >5.5 cm) or severe left ventricular dysfunction (i.e., left ventricular ejection fraction <30%). The primary endpoint evaluated will be freedom from recurrent AF over 1-year follow-up in the absence of AAD therapy. Among relevant secondary outcomes assessed, there will be left atrial and ventricular reverse remodeling and changes in symptom severity.

Cardioversion versus catheter ablation for persistent AF

The optimal treatment strategy for symptomatic persistent AF patients eligible for a rhythm-control therapy is still undefined. The aim of this trial is to compare external electric cardioversion plus AAD therapy versus catheter ablation in these patients. The study will evaluate important efficacy and safety endpoints. The primary efficacy endpoint will be freedom from recurrent AF at 6 months, as evaluated by 7-day HM. Total mortality, stroke, and incidence of PV stenosis will be among the safety endpoints assessed. The trial started on August 2005 and was estimated to finish on June 2009. Information on the current status of the study is not yet available.

References

1. Haïssaguerre M, Jaïs P, Shah DC, et al. Spontaneous initiation of atrial fibrillation by ectopic beats originating in the pulmonary veins. N Engl J Med 1998; 339:659–666.
2. Calkins H, Brugada J, Packer DL, et al. HRS/EHRA/ECAS expert Consensus Statement on catheter and surgical ablation of atrial fibrillation: Recommendations for personnel, policy, procedures and follow-up. A report of the Heart Rhythm Society (HRS) Task Force on catheter and surgical ablation of atrial fibrillation. Heart Rhythm 2007; 4:816–861.
3. Natale A, Raviele A, Arentz T, et al. Venice Chart international consensus document on atrial fibrillation ablation. J Cardiovasc Electrophysiol 2007; 18:560–580.
4. Camm AJ, Kirchhof P, Lip GYH, et al. Guidelines for the management of atrial fibrillation. Eur Heart J 2010; 31:2369–2429.
5. Wann LS, Curtis AB, January CT, et al. 2011 ACCF/AHA/HRS focused update on the management of patients with atrial fibrillation (updating the 2006 guideline): A report of the American College of Cardiology Foundation/American Heart Association Task Force on Practice Guidelines. Circulation 2011; 123:104–123.

6. Camm AJ, Kirchhof P, Lip GYH, et al. Guidelines for the management of atrial fibrillation. Europace 2010; 12:1360–1420.
7. Jaïs P, Cauchemez B, Macle L, et al. Catheter ablation versus antiarrhythmic drugs for atrial fibrillation: The A4 Study. Circulation 2008; 118:2498–2505.
8. Pappone C, Augello G, Sala S, et al. A randomized trial of circumferential pulmonary vein ablation versus antiarrhythmic drug therapy in paroxysmal atrial fibrillation: The APAF Study. J Am Coll Cardiol 2006; 48:2340–2347.
9. Wazni OM, Marrouche NF, Martin DO, et al. Radiofrequency ablation vs antiarrhythmic arugs as first-line treatment of symptomatic atrial fibrillation: A randomized trial. JAMA 2005; 293:2634–2640.
10. Wilber DJ, Pappone C, Neuzil P, et al. Comparison of antiarrhythmic drug therapy and radiofrequency catheter blation in patients with paroxysmal atrial fibrillation: A randomized controlled trial. JAMA 2010; 303:333–340.
11. Forleo G, Mantica M, De Luca L, et al. Catheter ablation of atrial fibrillation in patients with diabetes mellitus type 2: Results from a Randomized Study Comparing Pulmonary Vein Isolation Versus Antiarrhythmic Drug Therapy. J Cardiovas Electrophysiol 2009; 20:22–28.
12. Krittayaphong R, Raungrattanaamporn O, Bhuripanyo K, et al. A randomized clinical trial of the efficacy of radiofrequency catheter ablation and amiodarone in the treatment of symptomatic atrial fibrillation. J Med Assoc Thai 2003; 86:8–16.
13. Oral H, Pappone C, Chugh A, et al. Circumferential pulmonary-vein ablation for chronic atrial fibrillation. N Engl J Med 2006; 354:934–941.
14. Stabile G, Bertaglia E, Senatore G, et al. Catheter ablation treatment in patients with drug-refractory atrial fibrillation: A prospective, multi-centre, randomized, controlled study (Catheter Ablation For The Cure Of Atrial Fibrillation Study). Eur Heart J 2006; 27:216–221.
15. Calkins H, Brugada J, Packer DL, et al. HRS/EHRA/ECAS Expert Consensus Statement on Catheter and Surgical Ablation of Atrial Fibrillation: Recommendations for Personnel, Policy, Procedures and Follow-Up: A report of the Heart Rhythm Society (HRS) Task Force on Catheter and Surgical Ablation of Atrial Fibrillation Developed in partnership with the European Heart Rhythm Association (EHRA) and the European Cardiac Arrhythmia Society (ECAS); in collaboration with the American College of Cardiology (ACC), American Heart Association (AHA), and the Society of Thoracic Surgeons (STS). Endorsed and Approved by the governing bodies of the American College of Cardiology, the American Heart Association, the European Cardiac Arrhythmia Society, the European Heart Rhythm Association, the Society of Thoracic Surgeons, and the Heart Rhythm Society. Europace 2007; 9:335–379.
16. Calkins H, Reynolds MR, Spector P, et al. Treatment of atrial fibrillation with antiarrhythmic drugs or radiofrequency ablation: Two systematic literature reviews and meta-analyses. Circ Arrhythm Electrophysiol 2009; 2:349–361.
17. Nair GM, Nery PB, Diwakaramenon S, Healey JS, Connolly SJ, Morillo CA. A systematic review of randomized trials comparing radiofrequency ablation with antiarrhythmic medications in patients with atrial fibrillation. J Cardiovasc Electrophysiol 2009; 20:138–144.
18. Noheria A, Kumar A, Wylie JV, Jr., Josephson ME. Catheter ablation vs antiarrhythmic drug therapy for atrial fibrillation: A systematic review. Arch Intern Med 2008; 168:581–586.
19. Piccini JP, Lopes RD, Kong MH, Hasselblad V, Jackson K, Al-Khatib SM. Pulmonary vein isolation for the maintenance of sinus rhythm in patients with atrial fibrillation: A

meta-analysis of randomized, controlled trials. Circ Arrhythm Electrophysiol 2009; 2:626–633.

20. Rodgers M, McKenna C, Palmer S, et al. Curative catheter ablation in atrial fibrillation and typical atrial flutter: Systematic review and economic evaluation. Health Technol Assess 2008; 12:iii–iv, xi–xiii, 1–198.

21. Terasawa T, Balk EM, Chung M, et al. Systematic review: Comparative effectiveness of radiofrequency catheter ablation for atrial fibrillation. Ann Intern Med 2009; 151:191–202.

22. Pappone C, Rosanio S, Augello G, et al. Mortality, morbidity, and quality of life after circumferential pulmonary vein ablation for atrial fibrillation outcomes from a controlled nonrandomized long-term study. J Am Coll Cardiol 2003; 42:185–197.

23. Dagres N, Varounis C, Flevari P, et al. Mortality after catheter ablation for atrial fibrillation compared with antiarrhythmic drug therapy. A meta-analysis of randomized trials. Am Heart J 2009; 158:15–20.

24. Spragg D, Dalal D, Cheema A, et al. Complications of catheter ablation for atrial fibrillation: Incidence and predictors. J Cardiovas Electrophysiol 2008; 19:627–631.

25. Bubien RS, Knotts-Dolson SM, Plumb VJ, Kay GN. Effect of radiofrequency catheter ablation on health-related quality of life and activities of daily living in patients with recurrent arrhythmias. Circulation 1996; 94:1585–1591.

26. Spertus J, Dorian P, Bubien R, Lewis S, et al. Development and validation of the Atrial Fibrillation Effect on QualiTy-of-Life (AFEQT) Questionnaire in patients with atrial fibrillation. Circ Arrhythm Electrophysiol 2011; 4:15–25.

27. Dorian P, Cvitkovic SS, Kerr CR, et al. A novel, simple scale for assessing the symptom severity of atrial fibrillation at the bedside: The CCS-SAF scale. Can J Cardiol 2006; 22:383–386.

28. Kirchhof P, Auricchio A, Bax J, et al. Outcome parameters for trials in atrial fibrillation: Executive summary: Recommendations from a consensus conference organized by the German Atrial Fibrillation Competence NETwork (AFNET) and the European Heart Rhythm Association (EHRA). Eur Heart J 2007; 28:2803–2817.

29. Connolly SJ, Sheldon R, Thorpe KE, et al. Pacemaker therapy for prevention of syncope in patients with recurrent severe vasovagal syncope: Second Vasovagal Pacemaker Study (VPS II): A randomized trial. JAMA 2003; 289:2224–2229.

30. Catheter Ablation Versus Anti-arrhythmic Drug Therapy for Atrial Fibrillation Trial (CABANA). http://www.clinicaltrials.gov/ct2/show/NCT00911508?term=CABANA&rank=1. Accessed on January 2011.

31. Schotten U, Verheule S, Kirchhof P, Goette A. Pathophysiological mechanisms of atrial fibrillation: A translational appraisal. Physiol Rev 2011; 91:265–325.

32. Benjamin EJ, Levy D, Vaziri SM, D'Agostino RB, Belanger AJ, Wolf PA. Independent risk factors for atrial fibrillation in a population-based cohort. The Framingham Heart Study. JAMA 1994; 271:840–844.

33. Corley SD, Epstein AE, DiMarco JP, et al. Relationships between sinus rhythm, treatment, and survival in the Atrial Fibrillation Follow-Up Investigation of Rhythm Management (AFFIRM) Study. Circulation 2004; 109:1509–1513.

34. Kirchhof P. Can we improve outcomes in atrial fibrillation patients by early therapy? BMC Med 2009; 7:72.

35. Kirchhof P, Bax J, Blomstrom-Lundquist C, et al. Early and comprehensive management of atrial fibrillation: Executive summary of the proceedings from the 2nd AFNET-EHRA consensus conference 'research perspectives in AF'. Eur Heart J 2009; 30:2969–2977c.

36. Cosio FG, Aliot E, Botto GL, et al. Delayed rhythm control of atrial fibrillation may be a cause of failure to prevent recurrences: Reasons for change to active antiarrhythmic treatment at the time of the first detected episode. Europace 2008; 10:21–27.
37. van Gelder IC, Haegeli L, Brandes A, et al. Rationale and current perspective for early rhythm control therapy in atrial fibrillation. Europace 2011; in press.
38. Hsu LF, Jais P, Sanders P, et al. Catheter ablation for atrial fibrillation in congestive heart failure. N Engl J Med 2004; 351:2373–2383.
39. Khan MN, Jaïs P, Cummings J, et al. Pulmonary-vein isolation for atrial fibrillation in patients with heart failure. N Engl J Med 2008; 359:1778–1785.
40. Gasparini M, Auricchio A, Metra M, et al. Long-term survival in patients undergoing cardiac resynchronization therapy: The importance of performing atrio-ventricular junction ablation in patients with permanent atrial fibrillation. Eur Heart J 2008; 29:1644–1652.
41. Di Biase L, Mohanty P, Raviele A, et al. Preliminary results from AATAC: Ablation vs amiodarone for the treatment of persistent and long standing persistent atrial fibrillation in patients with congestive heart failure. Circulation 2010; 122:A17358.
42. Roy D, Talajic M, Nattel S, et al. Rhythm control versus rate control for atrial fibrillation and heart failure. N Engl J Med 2008; 358:2667–77.

CHAPTER 11

Surgical approach/ablation

Ralph Damiano Jr.[1], Stefano Benussi[2], Young-Hoon Kim[3], Jos G. Maessen[4], Helmut Mair[5], Domenico Mangino[6], Kalyanam Shivkumar[7], James R. Edgerton[8]

[1]Cardiothoracic Surgery Department, Washington University in St. Louis-School of Medicine, St. Louis, MO, USA
[2]Cardiac Surgery Department, San Raffaele Hospital, Milan, Italy
[3]Cardiology and Electrophysiology Department, Korea University Medical Center, Seoul, South Korea
[4]Cardiothoracic Surgery Department, University of Maastricht, Maastricht, The Netherlands
[5]Cardiac Surgery Department, University of Munich, Munich, Germany
[6]Cardiovascular Department, Dell'Angelo Hospital, Venice-Mestre, Italy
[7]UCLA Cardiac Arrhythmia Center, David Geffen School of Medicine at UCLA, Los Angeles, CA, USA
[8]Cardiothoracic Surgery Department, The Heart Hospital, Dallas, TX, USA

The pharmacologic treatment of AF has many limitations and inherent associated risks. In symptomatic patients with AF, conventional AADs have had relatively poor efficacy and numerous side effects. Because of these shortcomings, interventional techniques have gained widespread acceptance. The interventional era began in the early 1980s with the introduction of surgical approaches for AF [1–3]. While a number of these procedures are no longer performed, the CMP, introduced in 1987, has achieved success in treating both the symptoms and thromboembolic complications of AF. This procedure is the gold standard for surgical approaches. The following sections describe the current state of surgical ablation for the treatment of AF.

Historical aspects

The first procedure designed specifically to eliminate AF was described in 1980. In the laboratory of Dr. James Cox at Duke University, the left atrial isolation procedure was developed, which confined AF to the LA, and aimed to restore the remainder of the heart to sinus rhythm [1]. By isolating the LA but allowing the RA and right ventricle to contract in synchrony, a normal,

Atrial Fibrillation Ablation, 2011 Update: The State of the Art based on the VeniceChart International Consensus Document, First Edition. Edited by Andrea Natale and Antonio Raviele.
© 2011 John Wiley & Sons, Ltd. Published 2011 by John Wiley & Sons, Ltd.

right-sided cardiac output was provided, effectively restoring cardiac hemo-dynamics. This procedure eliminated two of the three detrimental sequelae of AF: the irregular heartbeat and compromised hemodynamics. However, since the LA remained in fibrillation, it did not eliminate thromboembolic risk. This procedure was performed in a single patient, and never gained widespread clinical acceptance.

In 1985, Guiraudon developed the corridor procedure for the treatment of AF [2]. This operation isolated a strip of atrial septum harboring both the SA and AVN, allowing the SA node to drive both ventricles. This operation eliminated the irregular heartbeat associated with AF, but both atria either re-mained in fibrillation or developed their own asynchronous, intrinsic rhythm because they were isolated from the septal corridor. The corridor procedure, while performed in a number of patients, was eventually abandoned because it had no effect on the hemodynamic compromise or the risk of thromboem-bolism associated with AF.

In 1985, Dr. James Cox and associates described the first procedure that at-tempted to terminate AF [4]. Using a canine model, Cox's group found that a single long incision around both atria and down into the septum could termi-nate AF. The atrial transection procedure prevented the induction and main-tenance of AF or AFL in every canine that underwent the operation. Unfortu-nately, this procedure was not effective clinically and was abandoned.

Development of the CMP

After almost a decade of laboratory investigation under the direction of Dr. James Cox at Washington University in St. Louis, the CMP was first clinically utilized in 1987 [3,5,6]. The procedure was initially developed to interrupt atrial macroreentrant circuits, thereby eliminating the ability of the atrium to flutter or fibrillate (Figure 11.1). The CMP was different from its predecessors such as the corridor procedure by its ability to restore both AV synchrony and sinus rhythm, thus potentially reducing the risk of thromboembolism and stroke [7]. The original operation consisted of creating full thickness incisions across portions of both the right and left atria. These incisions were precisely placed to allow the sinoatrial node to drive impulse propagation throughout both atria. This allowed for activation of nearly all of the atrial contractile mass except for the posterior LA, thus preserving atrial transport in most patients [8].

The first two versions of this procedure required modification, due to the high incidence of pacemaker dependence after the maze I and the technical difficulty of the maze II. The maze III procedure also referred to as the "cut-and-sew" maze, soon became the gold standard for the surgical treatment of AF (Figure 11.2) [9]. In a long-term study of patients who underwent the CMP III at our institution, 97% of the patients at a mean late follow-up of 5.4 ± 2.9 years were free from symptomatic AF [10]. These excellent results were reproduced by other groups [11–13].

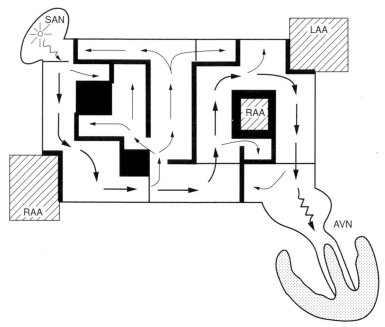

Figure 11.1 Schematic diagram of the maze procedure. (This article was published in The Journal of Thoracic and Cardiovascular Surgery, 101, Cox JL, Schuessler RB, D'Angostino HJ, et al. Surgical treatment of atrial fibrillation, 569–83. Copyright Elsevier, 1991).

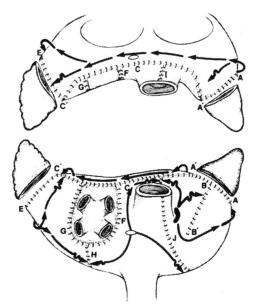

Figure 11.2 The lesion set of the Cox-maze III procedure. (This article was published in The Journal of Thoracic and Cardiovascular Surgery, 101, Cox JL, Schuessler RB, D'Angostino HJ, et al. Surgical treatment of atrial fibrillation, 584. Copyright Elsevier, 1991.)

The CMP III was effective in eliminating AF; however, it was technically difficult and invasive. With the introduction of ablation devices only a small number cardiac surgeons still perform the cut-and-sew operation today. Within the past decade, ablation devices have transformed the field of AF surgery by decreasing procedural difficulty and operative time, thus allowing for an application to a broader patient population and for the development of minimally invasive techniques [14].

Surgical ablation technology

Cryoablation

There are two commercially available sources of cryothermal energy that are being used in cardiac surgery. The older technology utilizes nitrous oxide and is manufactured by AtriCure (AtriCure, Inc., Cincinnati, Ohio). They provide both reusable and disposable probes. The disposable device has a 10-cm malleable probe on a 20 cm shaft. Medtronic (Minneapolis, Minnesota) distributes a newer device using argon technology. This technology uses either a malleable, single-use cryosurgical probe with an adjustable insulation sleeve or a two-in-one convertible device that incorporates a clamp and a surgical probe. At one atmosphere of pressure, nitrous oxide is capable of cooling tissue to $-89.5°C$, while argon has a minimum temperature of $-185.7°C$.

Cryoablation is unique among the presently available technologies, in that it destroys tissue by freezing instead of heating. The biggest advantage of this technology is its ability to preserve tissue architecture and collagen structure [14–16]. The nitrous oxide technology reliably creates transmural lesions on the arrested heart, and generally is safe, except around coronary arteries [17,18]. Argon-based technology has not been studied extensively. However, it appears to be able to reliably create endocardial transmural lesions on the arrested heart. Its ability to create epicardial transmural lesions on the beating heart is unclear, but available evidence suggests that it is unreliable in this setting [19]. Cryoablation has been shown to cause coronary injury, and its use should also be avoided near the esophagus [19]. Early clinical results have shown a good safety profile [20,21]. The potential disadvantage of this technology includes the relatively long time necessary to create an ablation (2–3 minutes). There also is difficulty in creating lesions in the beating heart, because of the heat sink of the circulating blood volume. The cryoclamp device may overcome this problem, as early work showed 93% transmurality on the beating heart [22]. However, if blood is frozen, it coagulates and may embolize. This may be a potential risk to epicardial cryoablation in this setting [14].

Unipolar RF energy

RF energy has been used for cardiac ablation for many years in the electrophysiology laboratory. It also was one of the first sources to be used in the operating room for AF ablation. It can be delivered by either unipolar or bipolar electrodes.

There are numerous unipolar devices in the market with the most popular technology distributed by Estech, Medtronic, and N-Contact. These have a variety of designs and configurations. They range from small, pen-like devices to long, flexible devices with multiple electrodes that utilize suction to maintain tissue contact. At the present time, most of the devices are irrigated. Unipolar RF devices have been shown to be able to create endocardial lesions effectively most of the time, but they have had difficulty creating reliable epicardial transmural lesions on the beating heart [23]. As with all unipolar energy sources, these devices radiate unfocused heat, and this has caused collateral injury when not used carefully. Complications of unipolar devices that have been described include coronary artery injuries, cerebral vascular accidents, and the creation of esophageal perforation leading to atrialesophageal fistulae [24–26].

To overcome some of the limitations of the unipolar devices, bipolar RF ablation was introduced. This technology has been incorporated into devices in two ways. The first is a clamp in which energy is applied between two embedded electrodes in the jaws of the device. The second way it is used is in devices in which the two electrodes are side-by-side and the device is applied to either the epicardial or endocardial surface of the atrium.

Three companies currently market bipolar RF clamp devices: AtriCure, Estech and Medtronic. With these devices, the electrodes are shielded from the circulating blood pool, allowing for faster ablation times and limiting collateral damage. Bipolar ablations have been shown to be capable of creating transmural lesions on the beating heart in animal models with short ablation times [27–29]. An advantage of bipolar RF energy is its safety profile. Despite widespread clinical use, there has been no collateral tissue damage described with bipolar RF technology.

The bipolar devices that utilize side-by-side electrodes have not been as reliable as the bipolar clamps in creating transmural lesions. The most widely used device was not capable of creating a linear line of conduction block on the beating heart in an animal model [23]. No studies have yet been done to determine the effect of multiple ablations at a single site.

High-intensity frequency ultrasound

HiFU is another modality that has been applied clinically for surgical ablation (St. Jude Medical, Minneapolis, Minnesota). HiFU is unique in that it is able to create noncontact focal ablation in a 3D volume without affecting intervening and surrounding tissue [30]. It uses ultrasound beams in the frequency range of 1–5 MHz or higher, creating focused lesions quickly by rapidly raising the temperature of the targeted tissue to above 80°C. Its ability to focus the target of ablation at specific depths is its major advantage over other energy modalities. Another advantage is its mechanism of thermal ablation. HiFU ablates tissue by directly heating the tissue in the acoustic focal volume, and is, therefore, much less affected by the heat sink of the circulating endocardial blood pool than unipolar or RF energy. While a few clinical studies using HiFU have shown encouraging early results, some centers have had disappointing outcomes [30–32]. The fixed depth of penetration of these lesions may be a major problem in pathologically thickened atrial tissue. Moreover, these devices are somewhat bulky and expensive to manufacture.

In summary, each ablation technology has its own advantages and disadvantages. It is imperative for surgeons to develop a complete understanding of the effects of each specific ablation technology on atrial hemodynamics, function, and electrophysiology. This will allow for more appropriate use of devices in the operating room. The inability to create reliable linear lesions on the beating heart remains a shortcoming of most devices and has impeded the development of minimally invasive, off-pump procedures, especially for patients with long-standing AF and large left atria. This has led to interest in hybrid procedures involving both epicardial and endocardial ablation in order not to leave any gaps in the ablation lines [33].

Indications

The indications for surgical ablation have been defined in a recent consensus statement [34] and include the following:

1 All symptomatic patients with documented AF undergoing other cardiac surgical procedures.

2 Selected asymptomatic patients with AF undergoing cardiac surgery in which the ablation can be performed with minimal risk in experienced centers.

3 Stand-alone AF should be considered for symptomatic patients with AF who either prefer a surgical approach, have failed one or more attempts at catheter ablation, or are not candidates for catheter ablation.

There is controversy regarding the referral of patients for surgery with medically refractory, symptomatic AF in lieu of less invasive catheter ablation. In our opinion, there are relative indications for surgery that were not included in the consensus statement. AF patients who develop a contraindication to long-term anticoagulation and have a high risk for stroke (CHADS$_2$ score $\geq$ 2) are excellent candidates for surgery. The CMP both eliminates AF in most of these patients, and also amputates the LAA. The stroke rate following the procedure off anticoagulation has been remarkably low, even in patients with high CHADS$_2$ scores [35]. Surgical treatment for AF also should be considered in patients with chronic AF who have suffered a cerebrovascular accident despite adequate anticoagulation. These patients are at high risk for repeat neurological events. In our series of over 200 patients with a stand-alone CMP, there was only one late stroke, and over 80% of patients were off anticoagulation at last follow-up [7,36]. Finally, symptomatic AF patients with a clot in the LAA who have failed medical therapy are not candidates for catheter ablation and should be referred for surgical ablation.

Surgical techniques and outcomes

There are a myriad of different surgical ablation procedures that are presently performed. They can be grouped into three broad categories that will be described as follow: the CMP, left atrial lesion sets, and PVI with or without ganglionectomy.

The Cox-maze procedure

The original cut-and-sew CMP III is only rarely performed today. At most centers, the surgical incisions have been replaced with lines of ablation using a variety of energy sources. The most widely adopted variation has been the CMP IV, which utilizes bipolar RF energy to replace most of the surgical incisions [37]. This RF ablation-assisted procedure incorporates most of the lesions of the Cox-maze III and is performed on cardiopulmonary bypass. The operation can be done either through a median sternotomy or a less-invasive right minithoracotomy [38]. The actual ablation pattern has been well described [37–39]. The PVs are isolated with the bipolar clamps on the beating heart. It is imperative to document entrance and/or exit block at the time of surgery. The right-sided lesion set is performed on the beating heart on bypass (Figure 11.3). The left atrial lesion set is performed via a standard left atriotomy (Figure 11.4).

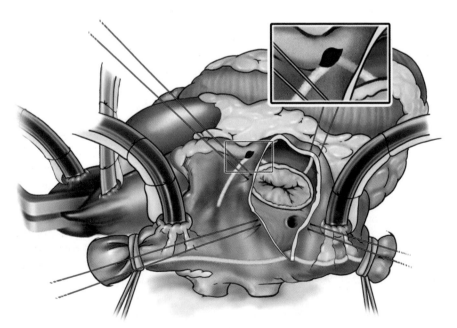

Figure 11.3 Right atrial lesion set of the Cox-maze IV procedure. (This article was published in The Journal of Thoracic and Cardiovascular Surgery, 141, Damiano RJ, Schwartz BA, Bailey MS, et al. The Cox Maze IV procedure: Predictors of late recurrence, 115. Copyright Elsevier, 2011.)

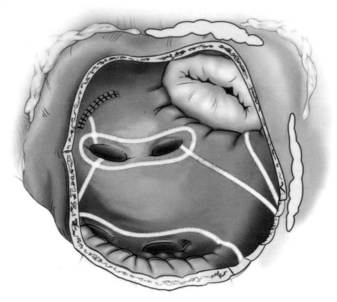

Figure 11.4 Left atrial lesion set of the Cox-maze IV procedure. (This article was published in The Journal of Thoracic and Cardiovascular Surgery, 141, Damiano RJ, Schwartz BA, Bailey MS, et al. The Cox Maze IV procedure: Predictors of late recurrence, 115. Copyright Elsevier, 2011.)

Outcomes

A propensity analysis performed by our group has shown that there was no significant difference in freedom from AF at 3, 6, or 12 months between the Cox-maze III and IV groups [40]. However, the CMP IV has significantly shortened operative times and lower complication rates. In our entire CMP IV series, the freedom from AF was 89% and the freedom from AF off AADs was 78% at 1 year [41]. In 100 patients undergoing a stand-alone CMP IV for lone AF, we reported a freedom from AF of 90% and freedom from AF off AA medication of 84% at 2 years with no intraoperative mortality and no postoperative strokes [42]. When patients ($n = 78$) isolation of the entire posterior LA with our current version of the Cox-maze IV, the freedom from AF at 12 months increased to 96%, with 86% of patients also free of AADs [42]. There was no difference in success rates for patients with paroxysmal compared with persistent or long-standing persistent AF.

PVI, expanded lesion sets, hybrid

The PVs have been isolated either separately or as a large box lesion incorporating the posterior LA. The first report of surgical PVI was in 2005. A bipolar RF clamp was used for PVI on the beating heart in 27 patients. At 3-month follow-up, 91% of patients were free from AF and 65% were off all AADs.

A larger series of a "box" isolation of all four PVs using epicardial microwave energy was performed endoscopically on the beating heart in

50 patients. Thirty-three patients had paroxysmal AF and 17 patients had continuous AF. At last follow-up, 79.5% of patients were in NSR. However, 27% of patients needed some type of late reintervention. The freedom from symptomatic AF and reintervention at last follow-up was only 49%. There was no operative mortality in either series.

Subsequent research confirmed that ablation of these triggering foci, while beneficial in the treatment of AF, entails significant recurrence rates. The contribution of the posterior LA is increasingly recognized as a source of non-PV triggering foci and as a substrate for maintaining AF. The posterior wall of the LA adjacent to the PV antrum has a shorter mean cycle length and greater number of discharges than other portions of the atrium [43]. Accordingly, electrophysiologists began to perform wide-antral encircling ablation that increased success [43]. In one study, circumferential PVI alone restored sinus rhythm in just 43.2% of patients with long-standing persistent AF [44]. In short, it has become increasingly evident that persistent (continuing for 7 days without termination) or long-standing persistent AF (e.g., "continuous"; defined as persistent AF for a year or longer) may not be successfully treated by PVI alone, since the mechanisms for initiation and maintenance of AF lie in the changed left atrial substrate beyond the PVs. From a pathophysiological perspective, this is explained by structural and electrical remodeling of the atrial myocardium, which can then initiate and sustain AF independent of the PVs in patients with persistent AF. In these patients, the augmented number and location of drivers for fibrillation necessitates additional linear ablation strategies, and sometimes multiple procedures with a commensurate shift toward posterior wall and LAA isolation. Indeed, the Cox-maze III emphasized the importance of right- and left-sided isthmus lesions, particularly of the left-sided isthmus, which includes ablation over the CS.

A number of studies support the contention that PVI alone is inadequate for persistent and long-standing persistent AF due to the substrate changes induced by electrical remodeling. Video-assisted bilateral PV antral isolation with confirmation of block and partial autonomic denervation was performed in 74 patients with follow-up at 6 months. A successful return to NSR for patients classified as persistent and long-standing persistent AF remained at 81.5% by ECG and dropped to only 56.5% by longer term monitoring [45]. In a larger study involving five surgical centers, 114 patients underwent the identical bilateral PV antral electrical isolation as in the prior study, with targeted autonomic denervation of the LA with selective left atrial appendectomy. Once again, the patients with persistent AF had a low success rate at 6-month follow-up, especially with longer term monitoring. NSR was found in only 18/32 (56.3%) of persistent cases, and only 11/22 (50%) of the long-standing patients [46].

Others have reported that long-term success of PVI is poor when compared directly with other lesion sets [47,48]. Such findings make clear that PV antral isolation and partial autonomic denervation are not adequate treatment in patients with persistent and long-standing persistent AF, with the associated changes in the left atrial substrate that occur in these conditions [49]. Because of electrical remodeling, the LA produces a shortened refractory period and a shortened fibrillatory interval [50]; atrial fibrosis may also be present [51]. It is apparent that elimination of the PV triggers alone is inadequate treatment for persistent and long-standing persistent AF. A more extensive lesion set, one that extends beyond PVI to include targets along the LA substrate, and one that can be performed epicardially on the beating heart, is necessitated.

The largest challenge to replicating the Cox-maze III lesion set on the full beating heart is making the connection to the mitral annulus. The other connecting lesions can be done through the transverse sinus. When connection lines to the mitral annulus are added, however, the success rates are shown to be comparable with the cut-and-sew maze: Jeanmart and colleagues reported an AF-free rate of 69.7% with an endocardial box lesion plus a connecting line to the mitral annulus [52]. However, incorporation of the MV isthmus can be challenging.

In traditional techniques, the connection to the MV is ablated across the left atrial isthmus. However, there are three inhibitors to doing this on the full beating heart. First, the traditional connection is to the posterior annulus, but visualization behind the full beating hearts' LA is very limited. Second, when working epicardial to endocardial, there is the risk of collateral damage to the circumflex coronary artery overlying the MV. Third, the CS, which is used as the epicardial landmark for the mitral annulus, is unreliable, and may leave a gap [53]. This leads to a significant risk of incomplete ablation or introducing AFL, because of reentry or electrical bridging by tissue [54–56].

To address these problems, the Dallas Lesion Set [57] was developed. The set replicates the left atrial lesions of the Cox-maze III. The problem of connecting to the MV is addressed by connecting to the anterior annulus at the left fibrous trigone. The MV touches the aortic valve at the left fibrous trigone that lies at the junction of the left and the noncoronary cusps of the aortic root. Thus an epicardial landmark is available [58], and visualization is excellent.

It interrupts conduction around the mitral annulus and is expected to interruption circuits causing left atrial tachycardias in other ablation procedures [59]. The other left atrial connecting lesions are done in the transverse sinus. A linear lesion is made from the RSPV to the LSPV and a line is made from the LSPV to the base of the amputated LAA. This completes all the left atrial lines of the Cox-maze III.

The operation is done with a bilateral thoracoscopic approach. The right side is approached first. A 5-mm port is placed in the right third or fourth ICS at the midaxillary line. CO_2 is insufflated to expand the thorax and aid in visualization. Two more 11-mm ports are placed. One is in about the second ICS at the midclavicular line and the other in about the sixth ICS at the midaxillary line. The pericardium is opened 2 cm anterior to the PN from top to diaphragm. Great care is taken at all times to protect the PN. Retraction sutures are placed in the posterior leaf of the pericardium and brought out through the posterolateral thorax. The SVC is then circumferentially dissected and rendered intrapericardial. Then the transverse sinus can be easily entered behind the PN. There is a very constant fat pad behind the SVC, on the dome of the LA. This must be divided. Fat is an insulator to RF energy and trying to burn through this fat will result in an incomplete lesion. Next a baseline map of the PV is taken. Then the bipolar RF clamp is placed around the PV antrum, well away from the bifurcation. Multiple firings are done after which the surgeon checks for entrance block. At his option, the surgeon may map for GP and ablate them. Attention is then directed to the transverse sinus. Using a bipolar directional RF pen, a line is made obliquely from the RSPV to the left fibrous triangle. The fibrous trigone is always hidden by loose areolar tissue that attaches the root of the aorta to the muscular dome of the atrium. Care must be taken to dissect down to the white fibrous trigone. Proper placement of the RF pen on the mitral annulus can be verified with the transesophageal echo using a mid-esophageal, long axis, 140-degree view. An oblique line is now made from the fibrous trigone up and away toward the LSPV. This line goes along the base of the atrial appendage. It will later be completed from the left side. Finally, a line is made from the RSPV to the LSPV in the transverse sinus. The right pericardium is closed, a soft silastic chest tube is placed, the lung is inflated and the ports are closed. Next mirror image exposure is obtained on the left side of the chest. This time the pericardium is opened behind the PN and no retraction sutures are placed. The ligament of Marshall is divided and baseline recordings of the PVs are made. Multiple firings of the bipolar clamp are done on the PV antrum and then the veins are checked for entrance block. Then again using the directional pen, the lines from the RSPV and the fibrous trigone are connected to the LSPV. This then leaves on the dome of the atrium an inverted triangle of viability. The surgeon can then check in this triangle for entrance block indication that the three sides of the triangle are complete. The LAA is now closed with an external clip or amputated with a stapler. The surgeon insures that the ablation lines extend to the base of the amputated appendage. A soft tube is placed, the port sites are closed and if the patient is not in normal rhythm, he is cardioverted.

The Dallas Lesion Set has been performed by only a small group of dedicated surgeons, and early results have been published on 30 patients with a mean age of 58 years [60]. The group included 10 patients with persistent, and 20 with long-standing AF. ECG, long-term monitoring and the use of AAD data were collected 6 months postoperative, and follow-up was 100%. Procedural related complications did not occur during follow-up, nor were there any deaths. Efficacy measured at 6 months was available for all patients, and showed a success rate indicated by the number of patients in sinus rhythm, of 90% in persistent AF patients, and 75% in long-standing persistent AF patients. The use of AADs was unnecessary in 78% of persistent, and 47% of long-standing persistent AF cases.

Further results of a multicenter registry including 124 patients showed less optimal safety assessment, but outcomes remained satisfactory. Operative mortality was only 0.8%, and procedure related complications were at a minimum of 10% (renal failure, pericarditis, pneumothorax, pleural effusion, reoperation for bleeding). Again, a high success rate was measured. After 6 months, NSR was achieved in 71–94%, depending on previous catheter ablation and measurement by ECG or long-term monitoring. One-year success rate obtained by long-term monitoring demonstrated a success rate of 63% in a group that had previously undergone catheter ablation ($n = 21$). Data by ECG even showed a success of 86% in patients who had not been ablated before. It can be concluded from these reported results that the Dallas Lesion Set is a safe procedure, and has a significant success rate in patients with paroxysmal, persistent, or long-standing persistent AF.

Further frontiers are likely to use hybrid approaches, combining the strengths of epicardial and endocardial ablation. One is more likely to be transmural when burning inside out and outside in simultaneously. The potential for improved outcomes through hybrid ablation also derives from combining expertise levels. Surgeons are very good at making linear lesions and electrophysiologists at mapping for completeness and "spot welding" gaps in lines. The demonstration of the efficacy of this approach awaits the completion of currently underway trials.

References

1. Williams JM, Ungerleider RM, Lofland GK, Cox JL. Left atrial isolation: New technique for the treatment of supraventricular arrhythmias. J Thorac Cardiovasc Surg 1980; 80:373–380.
2. Guiraudon GM, Campbell CS, Jones DL, et al. Combined sinoatrial node atrioventricular node isolation: A surgical alternative to His bundle ablation in patients with atrial fibrillation. Circulation 1985; 72:220.
3. Cox JL, Schuessler RB, D'Agostino HJ, Jr, et al. The surgical treatment of atrial fibrillation. III. Development of a definitive surgical procedure. J Thorac Cardiovasc Surg 1991; 101:569–583.
4. Smith PK, Holman WL, Cox JL. Surgical treatment of supraventricular tachyarrhythmias. Surg Clin North Am 1985; 65:553–570.
5. Cox JL. The surgical treatment of atrial fibrillation. IV. Surgical technique. J Thorac Cardiovasc Surg 1991; 101:584–592.
6. Cox JL, Canavan TE, Schuessler RB, et al. The surgical treatment of atrial fibrillation II. Intraoperative electrophysiologic mapping and description of the electrophysiological basis of atrial flutter and atrial fibrillation. J Thorac Cardiovasc Surg 1991; 101:406–426.
7. Cox JL, Ad N, Palazzo T. Impact of the maze procedure on the stroke rate in patients with atrial fibrillation. J Thorac Cardiovasc Surg 1999; 118:833–840.
8. Feinberg MS, Waggoner AD, Kater DM, Cox JL, Lindsay BD, Perez JE. Restoration of atrial function after the maze procedure for patients with atrial fibrillation. Assessment by Doppler echocardiography. Circulation 1994; 90:II285–292.
9. Cox JL, Boineau JP, Schuessler RB, Jaquiss RD, Lappas DG. Modification of the maze procedure for atrial flutter and atrial fibrillation. I. Rationale and surgical results. J Thorac Cardiovasc Surg 1995; 110:473–484.

10. Prasad SM, Maniar HS, Camillo CJ, et al. The Cox maze III procedure for atrial fibrilla-tion: Long-term efficacy in patients undergoing lone versus concomitant procedures. J Thorac Cardiovasc Surg 2003; 126:1822–1828.

11. McCarthy PM, Gillinov AM, Castle L, Chung M, Cosgrove D III. The Cox-maze proce-dure: The cleveland clinic experience. Semin Thorac Cardiovasc Surg 2000; 12:25–29.

12. Raanani E, Albage A, David TE, Yau TM, Armstrong S. The efficacy of the Cox/maze procedure combined with mitral valve surgery: A matched control study. Eur J Cardio-thorac Surg 2001; 19:438–442.

13. Schaff HV, Dearani JA, Daly RC, Orszulak TA, Danielson GK. Cox-maze procedure for atrial fibrillation: May Clinic experience. Semin Thorac Cardiovasc Surg 2000; 12:30–37.

14. Melby SJ, Lee AM, Damiano RJ. Advances in surgical ablation devices for atrial fib-rillation. In: Wang PJ ed. *New Arrhythmia Technologies*. Blackwell Futura: Oxford; 2005, pp. 233–241.

15. Lustgarten DL, Keane D, Ruskin J. Cryothermal ablation: Mechanism of tissue injury and current experience in the treatment of tachyarrhythmias. Prog Cardiovasc Dis 1999; 41:481–498.

16. Manasse E, Colombo P, Roncalli M, Gallotti R. Myocardial acute and chronic histological modifications induced by cryoablation. Eur J Cardiothorac Surg 2000; 17:339–340.

17. Mikat EM, Hackel DB, Harrison L, et al. Reaction of the myocardium and coronary ar-teries to cryosurgery. Lab Invest 1977; 37:632–641.

18. Holman WL, Ikeshita M. Ungerleider RM et al. Cryosurgery for cardiac arrhythmias: Acute and chronic effects on coronary arteries. Am J Cardiol 1983; 51:149–155.

19. Doll N, Kornherr P, Aupperle H, et al. Epicardial treatment of atrial fibrillation us-ing cryoablation in an acute off-pump sheep model. Thorac Cardiovasc Surg 2003; 51:267–273.

20. Mack CA, Milla F, Ko W, et al. Surgical treatment of atrial fibrillation using argon-based cryoablation during concomitant cardiac procedures. Circulation 2005; 112:I1–6.

21. Doll N, Kiaii BB, Fabricius AM, et al. Intraoperative left atrial ablation (for atrial fibril-lation) using a new argon cryocatheter: Early clinical experience. Ann Thorac Surg 2003; 76:1711–1715.

22. Milla F, Skubas N, Briggs WM, et al. Epicardial beating heart cryoablation using a novel argon-based cryoclamp and linear probe. J Thorac Cardiovasc Surg 2006; 13:403–411.

23. Schuessler RB, Lee AM, Melby SJ, et al. Animal studies of epicardial atrial ablation. Heart Rhythm 2009; 6:S41–S45.

24. Aupperle H, Doll N, Walther T, et al. Ablation of atrial fibrillation and esophageal in-jury: Effects of energy source and ablation technique. J Thorac Cardiovasc Surg 2005; 130:1549–1554.

25. Gillinov AM, Pettersson G, Rice TW. Esophageal injury during radiofrequency ablation for atrial fibrillation. J Thorac Cardiovasc Surg 2001; 122:1239–1240.

26. Demaria RG, Page P, Leung TK, et al. Surgical radiofrequency ablation induces coro-nary endothelial dysfunction in porcine coronary arteries. Eur J Cardiothorac Surg 2003; 23:277–282.

27. Prasad SM, Maniar HS, Diodato MD, et al. Physiological consequences of bipolar ra-diofrequency energy on the atria and pulmonary veins: A chronic animal study. Ann Thorac Surg 2003; 76:836–842.

28. Gaynor SL, Ishii Y, Diodato MD, et al. Successful performance of Cox-maze procedure on the beating heart using bipolar radiofrequency ablation: A feasibility study in animals. Ann Thorac Surg 2004; 78:1671–1677.

29. Melby SJ, Gaynor SL, Lubahn JG, et al. Efficacy and safety of right and left atrial ablations on the beating heart with irrigated bipolar radiofrequency energy: A long-term animal study. J Thorac Cardiovasc Surg 2006; 132:853–860.
30. Villamizar NR, Crow JH, Piacentino V, et al. Reproducibility of left atrial ablation with high-intensity focused ultrasound energy in a calf model. J Thorac Cardiovasc Surg 2010; 140:1381–1387.
31. Ninet J, Roques X, Seitelberger R, et al. Surgical ablation of atrial fibrillation with off-pump, epicardial, high-intensity focused ultrasound: Results of a multicenter trial. J Thorac Cardiovasc Surg 2005; 130:803–809.
32. McCarthy PM, Kruse J, Shalli S, et al. Where does atrial fibrillation surgery fail? Implications for increasing effectiveness of ablation. J Thorac Cardiovasc Surg 2010; 139:860–867.
33. Krul SPJ, Driessen AHG, van Boven WJ, et al. Thoracoscopic video-assisted pulmonary vein antrum isolation, ganglionated plexus ablation and periprocedural confirmation of ablation lesions. First results of a hybrid surgical-electrophysiological approach for atrial fibrillation. Circ Arrhythm Electrophysiol 2011; 4:262–270.
34. Calkins H, Brugada J, Packer DL, et al. HRS/EHRA/ECAS expert consensus statement on catheter and surgical ablation of atrial fibrillation: Recommendations for personnel, policy, procedures and follow-up. Heart Rhythm 2007; 4:816–861.
35. Pet MA, Damiano RJ Jr, Bailey MS, Moon MR, Lawton JS, Rinne AW. Late stroke following the Cox-maze procedure for atrial fibrillation: The impact of CHADS2 score on long-term outcomes. Heart Rhythm 2009; 6:S14.
36. Weimar T, Schena S, Bailey MS, et al. The Cox-maze procedure for lone atrial fibrillation: A single center experience over two decades. Circulation 2011. Submitted.
37. Gaynor SL, Diodato MD, Prasad SM, et al. A prospective, single-center clinical trial of a modified Cox maze procedure with bipolar radiofrequency ablation. J Thorac Cardiovasc Surg 2004; 128:535–542.
38. Lee AM, Clark K, Bailey MS, Aziz A, Schuessler RB, Damiano RJ Jr. A minimally invasive Cox-maze procedure. Operative technique and results. Innovations 2010; 5:281–286.
39. Damiano RJ Jr, Gaynor SL. Atrial fibrillation ablation during mitral valve surgery using the AtriCure device. Oper Tech Thorac Cardiovasc Surg 2004; 9:24–33.
40. Lall SC, Melby SJ, Voeller RK, et al. The effect of ablation technology on surgical outcomes after the Cox-maze procedure: A propensity analysis. J Thorac Cardiovasc Surg 2007; 133:389–396.
41. Damiano RJ Jr, Schwartz FH, Bailey MS, et al. The Cox maze IV procedure: Predictors of late recurrence. J Thorac Cardiovasc Surg 2011; 141:113–121.
42. Weimar T, Bailey MS, Watanabe Y, et al. The Cox-maze IV procedure for lone atrial fibrillation: A single center experience in 100 consecutive patients. J Interv Card Electrophyiol 2011; 31:47–54.
43. Wu TJ, Doshi RN, Huang HL, et al. Simultaneous biatrial computerized mapping during permanent atrial fibrillation in patients with organic heart disease. J Cardiovasc Electrophysiol 2002; 13:571–577.
44. Tilz RR, Chun KR, Schmidt B, et al. Catheter ablation of long-standing persistent atrial fibrillation: A lesson from circumferential pulmonary vein isolation. J Cardiovasc Electrophysiol 2010; 21:1085–1093.
45. Edgerton JR, Edgerton ZJ, Weaver T, et al. Minimally invasive pulmonary vein isolation and partial autonomic denervation for surgical treatment of atrial fibrillation. Ann Thorac Surg 2008; 86:35–39.

46. Edgerton JR, McClelland, JH, Duke D, et al. Minimally invasive surgical ablation of atrial fibrillation: Six-month results. J Thorac Cardiovasc Surg 2009; 138:109–114.
47. Gillinov AM, Bhavani S, Blackstone EH, et al. Surgery for permanent atrial fibrillation: Impact of patient factors and lesion set. Ann Thorac Surg 2006; 82:502–513.
48. Wisser W, Seebacher G, Fleck T, et al. Permanent chronic atrial fibrillation: Is pulmonary vein isolation alone enough? Ann Thorac Surg 2007; 84:1151–1157.
49. Gillinov AM, Bhavani S, Blackstone EH, et al. Surgery for permanent atrial fibrillation: Impact of patient factors and lesion set. Ann Thorac Surg 2006; 82:502–514.
50. Wijffels MC, Kirchhof CJ, Dorland R, Power J, Allessie MA. Electrical remodeling due to atrial fibrillation in chronically instrumented conscious goats: Roles of neurohumoral changes, ischemia, atrial stretch, and high rate of electrical activation. Circulation 1997; 96:3710–3720.
51. Nattel S, Shiroshita-Takeshita A, Cardin S, Pelletier P. Mechanisms of atrial remodeling and clinical relevance. Curr Opin Cardiol 2005; 20:21–25.
52. Jeanmart H, Casselman F, Beelen R, et al. Modified maze during endoscopic mitral valve surgery: The OLV clinic experience. Ann Thorac Surg 2006; 82:1765–1769.
53. Shinbane JS, Lesh MD, Stevenson WG, et al. Anatomic and electrophysiologic relation between the coronary sinus and mitral annulus: Implications for ablation of left-sided accessory pathways. Am Heart J 1998; 135:93–98.
54. Antz M, Otomo K, Arruda M, et al. Electrical conduction between the right atrium and the left atrium via the musculature of the coronary sinus. Circulation 1998; 98:1790–1795.
55. Cox JL. Atrial fibrillation II: Rationale for surgical treatment. J Thorac Cardiovasc Surg 2003; 126:1693–1699.
56. Jaïs P, Hocini M, Hsu L-F, et al. Technique and results of linear ablation at the mitral isthmus. Circulation 2004; 110:2996–3002.
57. Edgerton JR. Total thorascopic ablation of atrial fibrillation using the Dallas Lesion Set, partial autonomic denervation, and left atrial appendectomy. Oper Tech Thorac Cardiovasc Surg 2009; 14:224–242.
58. Edgerton JR, Jackman WM, Mack MJ. A new epicardial lesion set for minimal access left atrial maze: The Dallas lesion set. Ann Thorac Surg 2009; 88:1655–1657.
59. Lockwood D, Nakagawa H, Peyton MD, et al. Linear left atrial lesions in minimally invasive surgical ablation of persistent atrial fibrillation: Techniques for assessing conduction block across surgical lesions. Heart Rhythm 2009; 6:S50–63.
60. Edgerton JR, Jackman WR, Mahoney C, Mack MJ. Totally thorascopic surgical ablation of persistent AF and long-standing persistent atrial fibrillation using the "Dallas" lesion set. Heart Rhythm 2009; 6:S64–70.

CHAPTER 12

Hospital equipment and facilities, personnel, training requirements, and competences

Douglas L. Packer[1], Johannes Brachmann[2], Paolo Della Bella[3], Luc J. Jordaens[4], José L. Merino[5], Claudio Tondo[6], Gerhard Hindricks[7]

[1]Heart Rhythm Services, Mayo Clinic Health Systems/St. Mary's Hospital, Rochester, NY, USA
[2]Cardiology Department, II Med Klinik Klinikum Coburg, Coburg, Germany
[3]Cardiology Department, San Raffaele Hospital, Milan, Italy
[4]Thoraxcenter, Clinical Electrophysiology Department, Erasmus MC, Rotterdam, The Netherlands
[5]Cardiology Department, La Paz University Hospital, Madrid, Spain
[6]Arrhythmology Department, Centro Cardiologico Monzino, Milan, Italy
[7]Herzzentrum, Leitender Arzt Universität Leipzig, Leipzig, Germany

Hospital equipment, facilities, and technological requirements

Centers involved in AF ablation procedures should be equipped with state-of-the-art equipment. These should include the following:
• Sedation, anesthesia and resuscitation equipment, including pericardiocentesis materials, biphasic defibrillator and a mechanical ventilator. The long duration of the procedures and the potential serious complications of AF ablation make this equipment mandatory.
• Up-to-date ECG, blood pressure, oxygen saturation, and ACT monitoring equipment.
• Modern catheterization laboratories. Invasive electrophysiology procedures often expose both the patient and the operator to significant doses of radiation. This is especially true for AF procedures, which are among of the most irradiating. Therefore, all means to keep irradiation to the minimum and to follow the ALARA principle (as low as reasonably achievable) should be implemented, including X-ray systems allowing dose-reduction and image optimization and staff protection.

Atrial Fibrillation Ablation, 2011 Update: The State of the Art based on the VeniceChart International Consensus Document, First Edition. Edited by Andrea Natale and Antonio Raviele.
© 2011 John Wiley & Sons, Ltd. Published 2011 by John Wiley & Sons, Ltd.

- A multichannel recording system (at least a 16-channel recording system) and a multiprogrammable stimulator.
- 3D electroanatomical mapping: at least one system.
- RF power generators and/or cryoablation console.
- Cardiac imaging techniques. The center should have a cardiac imaging department, which should provide both transthoracic and transesophageal echocardiography. In addition, it is advisable that centers have access to a multislice-CT scanner or MR scanner to allow evaluation of coronary pathology and to reconstruct 3D anatomy of the LA and PVs.
- ICE availability is recommended although at present time the balance between the cost and added benefits of this equipment and its disposals on the procedure is unclear.

Other equipments, such as magnetic and robotic navigation systems and single-shot device systems, are promising but their impact and superiority compared to the conventional approach of AF ablation is unclear and remain speculative.

Training and knowledge

Indications and patient selection

Catheter ablation for AF has greatly evolved in the last few years, encompassing different approaches and new technologies. The primary goal of the procedure remains the improvement of QoL resulting from the amelioration of arrhythmia-related symptoms such as fatigue, palpitations, and effort intolerance. On the basis of this scenario, the main criterion of patient selection would be the occurrence of symptomatic AF. According to the current international guidelines, symptomatic patients could be considered adequate candidates for catheter ablation if refractory or intolerant to at least one class 1 or 3 AAD treatment. Specific attention should be paid also to patients with AF but asymptomatic and, with already documented inefficacy of at least one AA medication. This category of patients could be young and not fully committed to remain on long-term anticoagulation therapy and, therefore, they could be considered eligible for catheter ablation. In clinical practice, many young patients with symptomatic or asymptomatic AF seek catheter ablation because unwilling to continue long-term anticoagulation treatment with warfarin. This should not be portrayed as the rationale of performing catheter ablation, because patients should be aware that the arrhythmia may recur during the follow-up and the discontinuation of warfarin therapy depends on the clinical patient's characteristics (CHADS$_2$ or CHA$_2$DS$_2$-VAScscores) and not on patient's desire to eliminate a long-term anticoagulation therapy. The physician (i.e., electrophysiologist) should be competent in counseling patients and evaluating the potential risk and benefits of catheter ablation and should be able to direct current recommendations to the specific needs of individual patients.

Anatomical knowledge

Each electrophysiologist actively involved in AF ablation must have a detailed knowledge of cardiac anatomy with specific attention to LA and its adjacent structures. Excellence in cardiac anatomy is highly required for performing the technical aspects of TSP, cannulation of the LA, and navigation. The best knowledge of cardiac anatomy is also crucial to avoid or reduce the risk of procedure-related complications. Trainees in electrophysiology should be offered an intensive course on cardiac anatomy by an experienced pathologist as to easily recognize the anatomic relationship of the atria, SVC, and PVs to the pulmonary arteries, aorta, mitral annulus, PNs, sympathetic and parasympathetic innervation, esophagus and other mediastinal structures. The detailed knowledge of cardiac anatomy provides a unique occasion to appreciate also the myocardial tissue thickness of different atrial structures and, therefore, giving the operator the ability to adjust the energy used for ablation.

Interpretation of electrograms/knowledge in basic electrophysiological studies

Every electrophysiologist performing catheter ablation of AF must have achieved a proficiency in the ECG and intracavitary electrograms interpretation. Before ablating AF, trainees should have carried out a substantial number of supraventricular arrhythmias both in the RA and LA as to familiarize with intracavitary recordings and their correct interpretation. Furthermore, any pacing maneuvers aiming at making differential diagnosis among different cardiac arrhythmia disorders should be well mastered by any physician (trainee/attending/supervisor) involved in the AF ablation program. Proficiency in interpreting intracavitary recordings during AF ablation is of pivotal importance for understanding the endpoint of the procedure. Therefore, recognition of PV potentials both at baseline and during CS pacing and when PV electrical disconnection is achieved remains the cornerstone of the ablation procedure. With the evolving understanding of the pathophysiology of AF, especially for the persistent form of the arrhythmia, electrophysiologists are required to identify and interpret fractionated low-amplitude atrial potentials that, in accordance with published studies, may be equally considered target for ablation. The competence in mastering intracavitary recordings of supraventricular tachycardias is highly recommended, because these arrhythmias may act as trigger for AF and AFL and, therefore, the correct diagnosis is crucial, in these circumstances, for identifying the mechanism of AF.

Knowledge of 3D mapping systems

Catheter ablation of AF and atrial macroreentrant tachycardia necessitates accurate spatial anatomical and electrical orientation within a complex 3D substrate. Because of the limitations of 2D fluoroscopy to provide the required precision of 3D orientation, cardiac mapping systems have been developed to facilitate an accurate understanding of the electrical substrate within its anatomical boundaries. A realistic model of the individual 3D cardiac anatomy becomes even more important with introduction of anatomically guided ablation line placement, such as for the treatment of patients with AF. Any attempt of nonfluoroscopic intracardiac 3D orientation requires a technology for reliable, stable, and reproducible visualization and 3D localization of intracardiac catheters.

An electrophysiologist who performs AF ablation procedures must be familiar with the handling and interpretation, as well as with the limitations of different 3D mapping systems. Therefore, trainees should be able to perform and interpret the different types of electrophysiological analysis such as activation mapping for the treatment of left-atrial macroreentrant tachycardia, voltage mapping for substrate guided ablation approaches, and purely anatomical maps for conventional AF ablation procedures.

Technical competence

AF ablation is one of the most complex procedures of interventional electrophysiology. In addition to extensive knowledge of vascular and cardiac anatomy, signal interpretation, and 3D mapping mentioned above, technical competence and skills in catheter, sheath, and guidewire manipulation are required.

Basic technical skills
The trainee should be fully trained in simpler supraventricular tachycardia ablation procedures, including ectopic atrial tachycardia, AV nodal reentrant tachycardia, AV accessory pathways, and subeustachian AFL ablation. This includes proficiency in all aspects of the procedures depicted in Table 12.1.

Transseptal puncture
A good knowledge of TSP techniques is mandatory for all electrophysiologists involved in PV isolation, and other left-sided procedures [1,2]. Therefore, an understanding of the anatomy of the IAS is essential, with an insight in its relations with adjacent structures, as was mentioned above. A persistent oval fossa, which theoretically might make puncture redundant, is associated with

Table 12.1 Basic technical skills to be proficient for an AF procedure.

Vascular access and cannulation
Fluoroscopy system use and familiarity with fluoroscopic projections and landmarks
Catheter manipulation and positioning
Set up and understanding of the electrophysiology system, including the intracardiac recording system, the electrical stimulator, and the 3D electroanatomical system.
Knowledge on materials and systems to manage complications (defibrillator, pericardiocentesis kit, etc.)

more difficulties during PVI [3]. TSP for PV procedures should be relatively anterior to allow cannulation of the right-sided veins. Whether this remains necessary with magnetically steered catheters and flexible sheaths is not clear.

Fluoroscopic imaging techniques are useful as direct contrast imaging of the RA, rotational angiography of theLA, with the potential to document the overlapping area, and "tagging" of the oval fossa with contrast. Some investigators use additional anatomical landmarks such as a pigtail catheter in the aorta (which requires arterial puncture) or use His bundle or CS catheters as a reference. TEE andICE are great techniques to visualize the procedure online. ICE can be performed without general anesthesia. Echo helps to recognize other problems as clot formation, and aneurysmatic septa, with the danger of perforating the posterior wall. Further, ICE (and TEE) will help to prevent and manage complications [4].

Flushing of the sheaths and all material is necessary; air bubbles should be prevented. Standard Brockenbrough needles and sheaths are usually sufficient for ablation procedures. RF assisted TSP might be of additional value in thick or fibrotic tissue [5]. Once TSP is achieved, it is confirmed with contrast either on fluoroscopy or on echo; an alternative tool is recording of the pressure. Before puncture, heparin is administered; this is continued throughout the entire procedure, aiming at a high ACT (typically above 300 seconds).

Competence in performing basic electrophysiological studies and ablation procedures

The EHRA presently recommends receiving formal training for at least 1 year in conventional electrophysiology procedures and simpler ablations before being involved in AF ablation procedures [6]. Following this first year, the trainee should receive formal training in more complex procedures, one of them being AF ablation. According to this scientific organization, the trainee should be directly involved in a minimum number of 150 ablation procedures (35 to be performed as the primary operator) and 10 transseptal catheterizations (5 to be performed as the primary operator) at the end of this 2-year period. The Heart Rhythm Society Ad Hoc Committee on Catheter Ablation and the Canadian Cardiovascular Society Committee have recommended that a physician who performs catheter ablation procedures should have been the primary operator on 30 and 50 ablations, respectively [7]. The former committee also recommends involvement in 10 TSPs. The ACGME recommends involvement in a minimum of 75 catheter ablation procedures. However, these requirements are the basis to be trained in ablation procedures in general and possibly more practical experience, especially in transseptal catheterization, should be required to be fully competent to perform AF ablation procedures as independent operator and to manage potential complications, such as macroreentrant left atrial tachycardia [8]. To date, no scientific organization has established a minimum number of AF procedures to be performed as primary operator in order to be considered fully trained for this task by them. The ACC and the AHA recommend participation in 30–50 mentored AF ablations [7]. Anyhow, some reports suggested that results improved in center with experience in more than 100 AF ablations [9].

Management of complications

Complications during and after catheter ablation for AF are more frequent and more severe compared with other ablation procedures [10]. Trainees must be familiar with risk factors, clinical signs, and symptoms of potential early as well as delayed occurring complications. Thorough understanding of clinical patient history, risk factors as well as medical background, allergies, and baseline coagulation status are a prerequisite before starting a complex ablation procedure. During the procedure, attention should be paid to vital signs (blood pressure, heart rate, oxygen saturation) and possible "pops" as a sign of overheating during energy delivery. Hemodynamic deterioration should trigger conscious analysis of clinical signs of congestion or bleeding, fluoroscopic images, as well as performance of urgent TTE to exclude cardiac tamponade. Backup of an experienced physician with skills in emergency needle pericardiocentesis is necessary and training in pericardiocentesis definitely necessary. Knowledge of hospital structures for prompt access to cardiac surgery in case of emergency surgical procedures is needed. Awareness of risks of conscious sedation (including hypoventilation, aspiration, and respiratory arrest) as well as management of those should be trained.

Besides management of acute complications, recognition of delayed occurring complications is mandatory. This requires knowledge in typical symptoms of esophageal fistula, PV stenosis, or PN injury and the respective management strategies. The trainee should be familiar with typical provoking factors and preventive measurements of these complications.

Follow-up

The importance of adequate follow-up after AF catheter ablation arises from the complex nature of left atrial ablation procedures with potential delayed occurring severe complications as well as arrhythmia recurrences. Quality control can only be assessed if hospitals implement an organized structure to routinely assess data on outcome (complications, freedom from arrhythmia). Trainees must be familiar with the principles of adequate rhythm monitoring following AF catheter ablation with clinical trials necessitating more intense AF monitoring than in clinical practice [8,11]. They should be aware that it is very difficult to prove the absence of arrhythmias with a high degree of diagnostic accuracy due to the high incidence of asymptomatic episodes even in patients with previously highly symptomatic AF [12] and due to the reported unpredictable and at times very late (>12 months) occurrence of arrhythmia recurrences [13,14].

Competencies should be established concerning definition, frequency, characteristics, and risk factors of postprocedural atrial arrhythmias. The trainee must be familiar with indications and contraindications for cardioversion, concomitant AAD use, and timing of repeat ablation. Furthermore, the use of anticoagulation regimes must be set in the right context with adequate risk–benefit evaluation of thromboembolic and bleeding risks. Adequate risk stratification requires knowledge of the diagnostic accuracies of different monitoring strategies including the respective possibilities and limitations of noncontinuous and continuous rhythm monitoring devices.

References

1. Epstein LM. Nonfluoroscopic transseptal catheterization: Safety and efficacy of intracardiac echocardiographic guidance. J Cardiovasc Electrophysiol 1998; 9:625–630.
2. Lundqvist C. Transseptal left heart catheterization: A review of 278 studies. Clin Cardiol 1986; 9:21–26.
3. Knecht S. Impact of a patent foramen ovale on paroxysmal atrial fibrillation ablation. J Cardiovasc Electrophysiol 2008; 19:1236–1241.
4. Szili-Torok T. Transseptal left heart catheterisation guided by intracardiac echocardiography. Heart 2001; 86:E11.
5. Knecht S. Radiofrequency puncture of the fossa ovalis for resistant transseptal access. Circ Arrhythm Electrophysiol 2008; 1:169–174.
6. Merino JL. Core curriculum for the heart rhythm specialist. Europace 2009; 11:31–26.
7. Tracy CM. American College of Cardiology/American Heart Association 2006 update of the clinical competence statement on invasive electrophysiology studies, catheterablation, and cardioversion: A report of the American College of Cardiology/American Heart Association/American College of Physicians Task Force on Clinical Competence and Training developed in collaboration with the Heart Rhythm Society. J Am Coll Cardiol 2006; 3:1503–1517.
8. Calkins H, Brugada J, Packer DL, et al. HRS/EHRA/ECAS expert consensus statement on catheter and surgical ablation of atrial fibrillation: Recommendations for personnel, policy, procedures and follow-up. A report of the Heart Rhythm Society (HRS) Task Force on Catheter and Surgical Ablation of Atrial Fibrillation developed in partnership with the European Heart Rhythm Association (EHRA) and the European Cardiac Arrhythmia Society (ECAS); in collaboration with the American College of Cardiology (ACC), American Heart Association (AHA), and the Society of Thoracic Surgeons (STS). Endorsed and approved by the governing bodies of the American College of Cardiology, the American Heart Association, the European Cardiac Arrhythmia Society, the European Heart Rhythm Association, the Society of Thoracic Surgeons, and the Heart Rhythm Society. Europace 2007; 9:335–379.
9. Cappato R. Worldwide survey on the methods, efficacy, and safety of catheter ablation for human atrial fibrillation. Circulation 2005; 111:1100–1105.
10. Dagres N, Hindricks G, Kottkamp H, et al. Complications of atrial fibrillation ablation in a high-volume center in 1,000 procedures: Still cause for concern? J Cardiovasc Electrophysiol 2009; 20:1014–1019.
11. Kirchhof P, Auricchio A, Bax J, et al. Outcome parameters for trials in atrial fibrillation: Recommendations from a consensus conference organized by the German Atrial Fibrillation Competence NETwork and the European Heart Rhythm Association. Europace 2007; 9:1006–1023.

12. Hindricks G, Piorkowski C, Tanner H, et al. Perception of atrial fibrillation before and after radiofrequency catheter ablation: Relevance of asymptomatic arrhythmia recurrence. Circulation 2005; 112:307–313.

13. Mainigi SK, Sauer WH, Cooper JM, et al. Incidence and predictors of very late recurrence of atrial fibrillation after ablation. J Cardiovasc Electrophysiol 2007; 18:69–74.

14. Shah AN, Mittal S, Sichrovsky TC, et al. Long-term outcome following successful pulmonary vein isolation: Pattern and prediction of very late recurrence. J Cardiovasc Electrophysiol 2008; 19:661–667.

Index

Atrial Fibrillation Ablation, 2011 Update: The State of the Art based on the VeniceChart International Consensus Document, First Edition. Edited by Andrea Natale and Antonio Raviele.
© 2011 John Wiley & Sons, Ltd. Published 2011 by John Wiley & Sons, Ltd.